Best wishes
Jean Sutton

LET BIRTH BE BORN AGAIN!

REDISCOVERING & RECLAIMING OUR MIDWIFERY HERITAGE

By JEAN SUTTON
NZ R. G. O. N.   Reg. Midwife
Cert. Adult Education

ISBN 0-9541631-0-9
Copyright @ 2001 Birth Concepts UK

**Published by Birth Concepts UK
95 Beech Rd, Bedfont, Middx TW14 8AJ
United Kingdom.**

Printed by Sarsen Press.

Dedication

Dedicated to all those families with whom I have been privileged to share, "The Everyday Miracle" and who have taught me to look closely at, and re-assess everything I think I know.

To the many, many people with whom I have studied, or worked, laughed and cried during a lifetime of involvement with the "Birth Process".

Acknowledgements

Love and thanks to Bill, my longsuffering husband, who has always believed in me and never failed to encourage and support me through the long journey that is undertaken when writing a book.

Special thanks to my son and daughter-in-law, Rob & Julie, for looking after me during all my "working holidays" in Europe. Thanks for organising me so that I can share this vital lost wisdom with so many at conferences and study days. Particular thanks for all the hours spent editing, typesetting and producing this book. It has certainly been a team effort!

Thanks also - to Sue Pocock, illustrator extraordinaire! (Sue
you know more about birth now than you ever
thought you would!)
- to Pauline Scott, Alice Coyle and Jo Hindley
whose support and encouragement in the early
days was so valuable.

Finally, thanks to my grandaughter Deborah – a child who proves all this "stuff" I work so hard to communicate is worthwhile!

CONTENTS

I

Abbreviations And Terms Used In This Book

O.A	Occipito anterior. A baby head down with his back between mother' s hip and umbilicus.
L.O.A	Left occipito anterior. A baby on mother' s left side.
R.O.A	Right occipito anterior. A baby on mother' s right side.
O.P	Occipito posterior. A baby head down with his back between mother' s spine and hip bone
L.O.P	Left occipito posterior.
R.O.P	Right occipito posterior.
O.L	Occipito lateral.
O.L-A	Occipito lateral – anterior.
L.O.L – A	Left occipito lateral – anterior.
R.O.L	Right occipito lateral.
R.O.L – P	Right occipito lateral – posterior.
A.P	Anterior – posterior.

Spines	Ischial spines. Protuberances on either side of the pelvis forming the lower edge of the cavity.
A.R.M	Artificial rupture of membranes.
S.R.M	Spontaneous rupture of membranes.
Left Lateral	Side lying position assumed by mother when in bed that is neither helpful or hindering to the baby and uterus.
Foetus	The spelling is deliberate. "Foetus" is the original Latin.
"G" Spot	Nerve plexus at junction of bladder and urethra. Corresponds to male prostate gland.
Rhombus of Michaelis	Kite shaped area at the base of spine that includes the lower lumbar vertebrae plus the sacrum and coccyx.
Folding	Movement of baby's skull bones during birth where bones overlap at sutures.
Moulding	Alteration of shape of skull bones, esp. parietals to reduce skull diameter.
V.E	Vaginal examination.

Introduction

*"Let's restore birth to its rightful place as the safe,
simple and exciting family event it can and should be!"*

Welcome to this small book, in which I have tried to describe and
share much of the common sense wisdom that I have learned and
others have shared with me during an interesting and varied life.
Many of these people are no longer in practice, and were never
encouraged to record what they had learned " on the job " and been
able to test as they worked. Research didn't suddenly emerge during
the 1980's, but has always been part of successful midwifery care.

How often as midwives, are we faced with a problem that we feel
we should be able to fix, but for which we can find no help in our
books or protocols?

What do we say, when during the antenatal period we meet a woman
who is certain that she is going to have the perfect birth, but who is
obviously going to have "the works"? How can we help her change
things to increase the chances of her achieving what she expects?

What can we do for the mother desperate from the pain and lack of
sleep caused by an occipito posterior (OP) baby trying to rotate and
engage his head?

Where do we look for ideas when the dreaded words "post mature"
are uttered?

Once labour starts, how often do we feel helpless to offer anything
more than pain relief and patience, until the inevitable happens, and
ventouse, forceps or caesarian section end the torment? Soft lights,

music and back-rubbing will not influence the baby's progress through the mother's pelvis. Syntocinon may help, but at what cost to the contents of the baby's head?

Why are so many women finding themselves undermined in the one purely female area of life? The amount of postpartum morbidity and depression seems to have increased despite our efforts.

How did we come to be seduced by desire to extend the role of the midwife into becoming the very good obstetric nurses so many of us are?

Where is the research into midwifery rather than medical aspects of birth?

This little handbook has been written for practising midwives, who are finding it hard to accept that the human birth process is designed to cause so many problems. Common sense tells us that if it had always been so, the human race would be as extinct as the dodo. In today's Western society, if there was not the extensive technical help, large numbers of babies, and probably their mothers too would be lost during birth. What's gone wrong?

In this book, an attempt is made to trace the original plans, by studying the relationship between the mother and her unborn. This covers the physical relationship, or anatomy and physiology of their interaction. It also looks at the way the baby has been changing his mother from the time he was the size of a pinhead until his final entrance to the world. We have no difficulty accepting the amazing changes of pregnancy, so why do we find it so hard to believe that the baby has a major influence on the way he is born?

Today there is a great deal of talk about the midwifery or social model of birth as opposed to the medical model. For many women though, there is no real choice. If her baby is to be born, it needs the help of technology. A baby overdue, and presenting in an awkward position, has a hard path ahead unless the mother's care-givers are able to provide suitable help.

As we travel together through this book it is my hope that we will find answers to many of those problems that currently make midwifery so stressful. Let's restore birth to its rightful place as the safe, simple, and exciting family event it can and should be, (for most women), where the midwife is the primary care-giver, and technology is kept in its place for the few women and babies who need it. Let the birthplace once again be a place of celebration of new life, rather than the intensive care unit it has become!

Many ideas will be repeated at intervals and in varying forms. This is deliberate, as many things written conflict with what we have been taught, though most of us will realise that they make clear what our senses have been recording. There is a great deal of misunderstanding of the normal process being taught as fact.

Most women, mothers and midwives have deep inside them the "women's wisdom" of generations gone before. It tells us that what is happening is not right, and makes us uncomfortable as we carry out the protocols laid down for us. We feel that there must be better ways to help, but can't quite define them. Once we have really understood how birth should happen, we will feel more confident about providing total care, antenatally, during parturition, and very importantly, postnatally.

The knowledge we need is available, written in old midwifery textbooks, and there are still some people with the "hands on skills". Soon it will be too late to ask that night Sister who solves so many problems how she does it.

Our greatest support will come from the mothers who have had our support and care throughout their "everyday miracle" as well as their partners and other support people.

This book is not anti-technology. In many of the situations that arise today we need all the help we can find. Pre-existing complications and medical problems are also beyond the scope of this book, as are difficulties such as placenta praevia. It is about providing midwifery skills that will help us give maximum assistance to mothers with vertex presentations. It is designed to help practising midwives assess more clearly just what each baby is trying to do and thus provide the maximum chance for the mother to achieve the birth she is hoping and planning for. Today, many women have a birth plan that is simply unrealistic, but if we are able to give her and the midwives the knowledge they need, she and her baby will be able to work together to make it possible.

If we look at the female pelvis and the foetal head from an engineering angle, we will see quite quickly how to help. There is no magic anywhere, although after helping some-one who had had four forceps deliveries and the fifth a caesarian manage not one, but two normal births it would be easy to believe there was. *The seventh was to prove the sixth wasn't a fluke.*

It is accepted in the following pages that the baby has his own role to play in a successful birth. He is not a passive recipient of outside forces. We know that he is an active individual during the pregnancy, so why is it so hard to believe that he is still an active participant throughout the birthing process? Modern research is finding that foetal or placental hormones trigger most of the processes of pregnancy and birth. (Professor Liggins of Auckland has done much study among animals and his results can be applied to humans).

It is also accepted that;

- When given the information they need, most women will produce realistic plans for birth.
- If the situation cannot be resolved within a reasonable time frame, appropriate intervention will be provided without subjecting the birthing couple to prolonged hopeful treatments.

(A cervix dilated to 5cm, with no increase for a couple of hours, and a baby lying R O L-P is a recipe for caesarian section, not syntocinon. Unless the baby can be persuaded to move, the situation is unlikely to improve.)

With all these maxims in mind, I hope that you will both enjoy and learn from the following pages and that your ensuing practise will continue to become ever more enlightened and satisfying as a result.

Let Birth Be Born Again!

Section One

An Overview Of
Normal Birth

Section One: An Overview of Normal Birth

"Successful reproduction or survival of the species is built into every living thing on the planet."

Modern Lifestyles and Their Effect on the Birth Process

Mankind was designed, or evolved, as a hunter - gatherer, travelling light, and over relatively long distances to find food and shelter. Men hunted live animals, and women spent hours digging for roots and tubers to add to their diet. During the seasons that fruits were ripening, stretching and bending to reach the best was also a woman's chore. Grain was harvested, again in a stooping position. Add to this the time she spent squatting to grind the grain and prepare the food and it is not hard to see that our foremothers had a very different life-style. Even when she rested, there was no furniture for sitting or sleeping, there was only the ground or a pile of animal skins.

As societies developed ways of producing or acquiring life's necessities, first tents, and then permanent homes became the norm. Despite this, women still needed to do many physical chores, to maintain their homes. Sweeping, floor washing, bending over a stream or tub to wash clothes, kept postures much the same. Chopping firewood, gardening or carrying water,- women were still very active.

Today, life is different for most women. Since the 1960's we have seen the introduction of television, and the design of "comfortable" lounge furniture. Washing machines, tumble dryers, dishwashers - all save women from physical effort. Even floormops save us from hand and knees cleaning!

Supermarkets too provide a wonderful variety of foods at all times of the year; meaning no need to grow and preserve as before.

Driving to work or to the shops may be faster, and it is certainly easier to fetch the groceries this way, but the walk to the local shops used to provide both exercise and an opportunity to spend time in an informal way with other women.

Another dramatic change came with the contraceptive pill and its ability to allow women to control their fertility.

The major drawback to today's lifestyle is the need for money to pay for what's available. Women need to go to work to help the family budget. Very few jobs involve physical activity, or are close enough to home to make walking or cycling an option. Getting to one's job may involve travelling long distances by car or bus. This is bad for anyone's back, as people are not designed to sit still, especially in cars where their knees are higher than their bottoms. This puts unnatural strain on the lower back.

Well-paid jobs require educated people. Thus girls are no longer able to be with women during the adolescent years, but spend most of their time with other girls the same age. Traditional "women's wisdom" was once passed from generation to generation, as new mothers were helped and supported by younger sisters or nieces. Girls grew up understanding what newborns needed. Grandmothers lived nearby and provided stability. All this has changed.

As family sizes decreased and more children started pre-school mothers went back to work. This further reduced the interaction between age groups where all the latest happenings were discussed.

Building new suburbs also meant that it was likely that all the children of a neighbourhood would be of similar age, and there were no babies to "practise" on. As mothers became even more protective of their fewer offspring, they forgot that the age when children best learn about baby care is between 10 and 12. Far too young to be trusted! Not so, the child is unlikely to be distracted by her own hormones at that stage.

Community midwives, who knew how each family functioned, and which ones were "good" birthers, became fewer, as the hospital roster system took them into a new role. Pregnant women were left to get their help from overworked and understaffed clinics, or lay teachers. As their textbooks are no different from ours, the basic understanding of the process of birth has been lost.

Many of these classes and books raise women's hopes to a level that is hard to achieve even when all goes well. They tend to forget that there is a second person involved in the birth process, and though we can see him by scan, we still can't communicate with him.

Perhaps we midwives should have guarded the responsibility for antenatal education more strenuously? Doctors, physiotherapists and lay teachers all have a role to play in complete mother/baby care, but we are the only ones who follow the baby from 'Womb to World'.

We know how to interpret what the mother is saying about her baby's movements, and how to connect that information with our observations of the pregnancy and labour. We do most of the vaginal examinations during labour and know that a lot of things written in our books are not what our fingers feel.

<u>*The Normal Birth Process*</u>

"Birth is an involuntary process, and as such cannot be managed"
(Michel Odent; Hawaiian conference 1995).

Once the process of pregnancy and birth has begun, its sequence is automatic, unless or until efforts are made by so-called helpers to control it.

Successful reproduction, or survival of the species, is built into every living thing on the planet. Human babies are no exception. They come complete with a master plan for safe, straightforward birth. As we know, there are many obstacles along the way, but until around the 1960's at least 85% of those who grew to full term got the exit message right. -----that is, L O A (vertex left occipito-anterior). A multigravida's baby may choose R O A (right occipito-anterior).

About 5% are breech, which isn't too bad as long as the baby faces backwards, and his mother remains mobile. The occasional one chooses the oblique angle; or transverse sometimes if the mother has had lots of babies. Some had their placentas below them, and some had a twin or triplet to complicate the journey.

That left around 10% who chose Vertex R O P (vertex right occipito- posterior). It was a surprisingly small number. Of these, about half would sort themselves out on the way through the pelvis, so only 5% would need help. What a contrast to today !!!

While birth is a pre-destined event, how the birthing pair interacts can be influenced by a number of factors. Some of these are physical, some hormonal, but many are due to today's lifestyles.

The Effects of Changing Postures

(a)

Standing
Good Lordosis.
Mother upright & forward.
Plenty of space between spine
& symphasis.
Baby supported by mothers
abdominals.

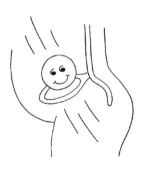

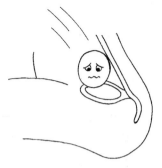

(b)

Sitting.
Little or no lordosis with baby in O.P
position.
Inlet level, preventing baby bringing his
back forward to allow head under the
sacrum.
MAY ENTER IN LABOUR

(c)

Squatting - Western women
bring spine forward & bottom
down, closing the inlet &
tightening the pelvic floor.
This is not advisable.

13

The Basic Design

We will look at the basic process, first from the mother's view, and then the baby's. Human mothers give birth easily if during the last few weeks of pregnancy they:

1. Help their baby achieve the Optimal Position (vertex L O A)

2. Concentrate their thoughts on the " every day miracle ".

3. Accept the physical and hormonal ripening of their body.

4. Adapt their postures to allow their baby to play his part in fitting through the pelvis---always keeping their weight in front of or above their ischial tuberosities (seat bones).

5. Understand that effective labour has begun only when their uterus changes shape with contractions.

6. Are aware that their cervix opens as an ellipse not a circle (see page 16), that is, the back remains in the same place, while the front stretches over the baby's head. That this is why the Braxton Hicks contractions have little or no effect with regard to opening the cervix. (It's just as well, as otherwise the baby would have fallen out weeks before).

7. Understand that their cervix does not lie in the middle of their vagina parallel to its sides, but is pointing towards the junction between sacrum and coccyx---even more posterior if their baby is not in the optimal position.

8. Realise that the pelvis is widest from side to side at the top. and from front to back at bottom. This means that the baby must make a 90° turn in the cavity. He enters with his face towards his mother's right side, and turns to face her spine.

9. Understand the importance of mobility during labour, so that they are able to respond to pressure from their baby's head. This decreases need for pain relief, and shortens the time for birth.

10. Understand that in most cases there will be a pause between first and second stage labour during which uterus and baby re-arrange themselves.

11. Realise that the back of their pelvis---the rhombus of Michaelis --must move backwards to open the pelvis to allow the baby out without deliberate pushing.

12. Are able to find something higher than waist level to grasp when the baby is ready to emerge.

13. Are able to open their knees, allow their body to sag, and arch their back as the baby emerges.

14. Remember to always make sure that the angle between their spine and thighs is more than 90°----no sitting back on their heels.

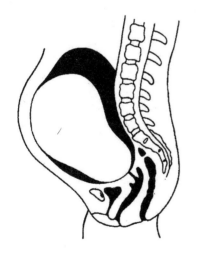

Primagravida's uterus at end of pregnancy

Cervix pointing correctly

How the Cervix Opens

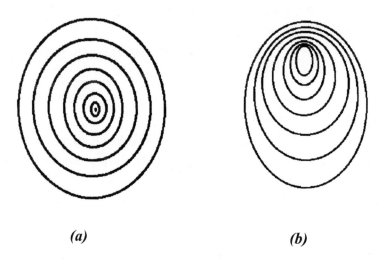

(a)   *(b)*

Cervix opening as circle   **Cervix opening as ellipse**
(wrong)   **(correct)**

See how the cervix really opens (b). It is behind the baby's head at the beginning and stretches forward with each contraction.

"The pain sweeps from the back to the front."

Direction of Contractional Force in O.A & O.P. baby

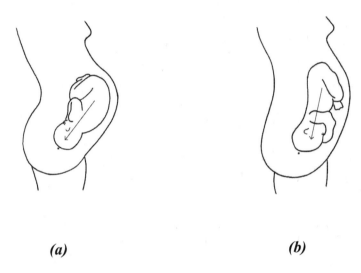

(a)   (b)

(a)   O.A - curls up and presses on cervix with each contraction

(b)   O.P - stays erect and pressure is on lower segment 2-3 cm in
       front of the cervix (wrong)

<u>Human Babies Birth Easily if They Follow The Master</u> <u>Plan</u> (the blueprint)

That is each one:

1. By term, lies head down on the mother's left side: between her hip and umbilicus, back forward and bottom pushing her abdominal muscles out. His head and body are at right angles to each other.

2. Turns its head towards the left 1/8th of a circle, bringing the right ear to the front, and facing directly right.

3. Begins to enter the mother's pelvis, slowly rotating head.

4. As labour starts and contractions bring his bottom further forward, bends head closer to chest, bringing face directly under mother's sacral prominence.

5. Near the end of first stage turns shoulders to right to lie across the pelvic inlet.

6. Has head and shoulders again at right angles to each other.

7. Brings bottom further forward to allow shoulders to enter pelvis as head leaves the uterus and enters the mother's vagina.

8. Presses "trigger" spot at base of mother's bladder--so-called G-spot--(see definition) to start second stage of labour.

9. Lifts his head and emerges into the world facing backwards.

10. Rotates head and body until right shoulder is against symphasis.

11. Allows anterior shoulder to rest against inside of symphasis.

12. Brings posterior shoulder (left) over the perineum.

13. Births anterior (right) shoulder.

14. Slides face down onto floor or bed.

15. Rests until placenta contracts.

16. Breathes, and waits to be lifted by mother.

17. Within a short time (this varies between babies) begins to "root" about ready to begin feeding.

When mother and baby co-operate in this process, it takes around 4 - 8 hours for a first baby, and about 2 - 4 hours for subsequent ones.

The babies come into the world peaceful and relaxed, looking about them with wide eyes. The mothers are able to manage with little or no outside assistance, have an intact perineum, and after a cup of tea, shower and sleep, progress through the next stage of adaptation to motherhood very easily.

The satisfying feeling of "I did it myself" carries them safely through the rough patches of the early postnatal days. Breast feeding usually proceeds smoothly, as the mother is able to concentrate on the baby, rather than the difficulties of finding a comfortable position. There is none of the physical distress from a painful, bruised, swollen and sutured pelvic area to impede the pleasure of becoming a parent.

We will now look at the whole process in more detail.

<u>Normal Birthing</u>

Full term baby
Uterus low
Cervix pointing in correct direction

L.O.A

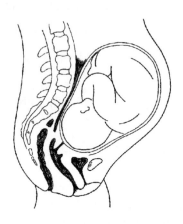

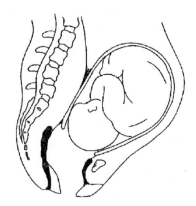

Full dilation before engagement

Note position of posterior lip

Engagement and rotation complete

Note nose against top of sacrum

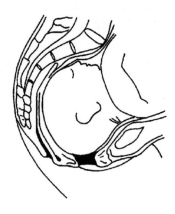

Preparing For Birth

During the last few weeks of pregnancy, the mother and baby have specific actions to take if the birth process is to begin on time, and proceed smoothly. The baby will do his part automatically, if the mother provides the right internal environment.

By around 36 / 40 weeks gestation, the baby takes up more room than the liquor. At this stage he ceases to be "weightless "---the mother now feels her body quite differently. Until now, she has been growing bulky and increasingly awkward, but the baby has not been felt as a separate entity. Suddenly this changes, and the baby can be felt as an object, though at all times he remains buoyant and able to move freely. Now the mother must accept that her body is ready to begin preparations for labour. As her hormones soften the tissues of her pelvic area, her back will curve further with the lordosis of pregnancy. This brings the uterus forward, and increases the angle between the sacral prominence and the symphasis.

In the primagravida's pear shaped uterus the baby *must* lie on the mother's left, which she also should try to do. If the baby is lying on his mother's right, he will feel unstable when she lies on her left. She should place a flattish pillow under her uterus to give him a little support, while still allowing him to turn. Later babies are in an apple shaped home, and may choose left or right.

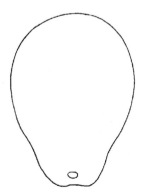

Pear shaped primigravida's uterus.
(Back View)

Clearly shows cervix at back of uterus.

21

Nature goes to great lengths to help babies make the best choice!

From this position, baby gives his mother's body very clear signals.

Her birth passage tissues relax, and become swollen and stretchy. Her cervix shortens and softens, ready to dilate easily. The pelvic ligaments become even more relaxed, so the mother's lower body may feel very uncomfortable. At this stage a maternity girdle may give comfort.

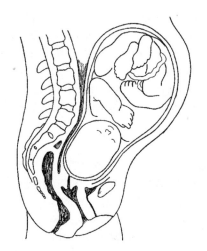

Usual version of full term baby. Cervix in midline (wrong)

This is the picture most mothers see.

It wrongly shows the cervix lying at the same angle as the vaginal walls.

Birthday

Once our baby has been persuaded to tuck himself up properly, that is, on his mother's left, with his back between her hipbone and umbilicus, he is ready for his journey to the outside world.

Unfortunately, many modern practices introduced to facilitate obstetric care have deprived women of the opportunity to utilise gravity and mobility in labour.

Practices developed without a sound understanding of the anatomy and physiology of the normal have caused a whole generation of women totally unnecessary harm.

With baby engaged L O A, labour begins smoothly, and progresses steadily. The early contractions are short, sharp, and well spaced. The uterus changes its shape with them; "rearing up" is the textbook's term. This obviously only applies if the mother is bedridden. If the mother is able to just bend forward, all the energy is available to hasten progress. Mothers need to know that labour is not established until the uterus changes shape with each contraction.

To provide adequate space a woman must either remain on her feet, or sit on her ischial tuberosities. This requires an angle that keeps her knees lower than her seat, and her lower legs dangling. This position cannot be achieved while sitting in bed! It is the one assumed when sitting on a toilet. (No wonder so many mothers want to stay there!) With his mother in this posture, the baby, if not already engaged, enters the brim in the optimal position. This position also increases pressure on the cervix.

The baby is able to bend his head further into the sacral curve until his face is directly under the sacrum. Then his shoulders are able to easily rotate to the direct transverse as they enter the pelvic brim. He is now a very compact little parcel. Contractions become closer, longer, and stronger as labour progresses.

Soon the very strong powerful contractions of transition occur, as first stage nears its end. This part of labour is harder to cope with, but the mother should be well into her abstracted, self centred, timeless, endorphin stage, if no-one is distracting her.

The "Rest and be Thankful" Stage

As first stage labour ends, and the membranes rupture there will usually be a short pause. For primigravida it may be quite long, up to half an hour, but for multigravida it varies from a few seconds to around five (5) minutes. Some mothers may even have a short sleep at this point.

During this time, the uterine muscle readjusts itself following the sudden decrease in internal tension caused by the loss of liquor, and the baby's head leaving the uterus and entering the vagina. The baby makes his final moves into the direct A P diameter---that is, he is now facing his mother's spine. His shoulders should be straight across the inside of the pelvic brim. This is very important--he can't descend if his anterior shoulder is sitting on the brim!! Remember; we are discussing a baby who began his journey as an O A.

Second stage now begins----

We need to recognise that just because a mother's cervix is "fully dilated" it does not mean that she is in second stage. For it to proceed smoothly, the baby *must* have finished rotating his shoulders into the transverse. Until then his head is unable to move down. (Think of the many small babies whose mothers push for ages, and who are delivered by ventouse).

It is important that the mother remains in an upright position. If standing, she must have something solid and higher than her waist to hold. Kneeling, she must bring her arms up also. Failure to do this will almost always result in the mother moving her weight backwards and actively pushing. This will put excessive pressure too far back on the perineum and cause a nasty tear. The same thing happens if the mother is trying to give birth while in a deep squatting posture. If a birth stool is used, it should be high enough to keep the mother's knees lower than her seat. If she is unable to, a compromise is the left lateral position, but *never any dorsal position.*

There should be *no pushing* needed. The baby is descending as the contractions change their character, and become expulsive. The back of his neck presses against the area of the maternal pelvis known as the G-spot. This corresponds to the male prostate gland, and is at the junction of the bladder and urethra. Nerves of both systems supply it. In the voluntary system the pelvic plexus of the inferior hypo-gastric nerve and the clitoral nerve supplies it. In the involuntary system, the supply is from the pelvic splanchnic system. With further investigation, we may find other nerves involved.

The effect of this pressure is to trigger a whole set of exciting events.

The mother's rhombus (that area of her spine including the sacrum and three lower lumbar vertebrae) moves backwards up to 2cm. As it does so, it pushes the wings of the ilia outwards. Jamaican midwives described this sequence to Sheila Kitzenger as "the mother opening her back ".

The mother reaches upward to find something above waist level to grasp. She allows her body to sag and her knees to rotate outwards.

Now comes the "foetal ejection reflex" described by Michel Odent.

The mother moves her body, often thrusting her hips forward and the baby begins to emerge.

He should do this very quickly, as he is in front of, not on the pelvic floor---the mother's spine lifts out of his way, and her coccyx is further up her body than her pubes as her back arches. His head is out, his shoulders rotate into the A P diameter, descend, and the anterior fixes against the mother's pubes as his posterior shoulder is born. Now he brings his anterior shoulder out, and lies face down on the floor, mat or bed.

If allowed to happen in this way, the baby doesn't need "delivering." In fact, less than five per cent (5 %) will need help.

Being born face down is an important survival move. Any secretions will be able to drain from his nose or mouth before he tries to breathe. For most babies, this does not happen instantly. He is quite safe, as his cord will still be pulsating and keeping him well. The normal scene has the baby sneezing before his first breath, which again clears any rubbish. Unless he is too cold he may not move until his placenta begins to detach. Once again, this is rarely instantly, as the mother's uterus must again respond to the loss of contents, and falling hormone levels.

The Posterior Shoulder is Born First!

The anterior shoulder (**x**) is seen first but the posterior is born first.

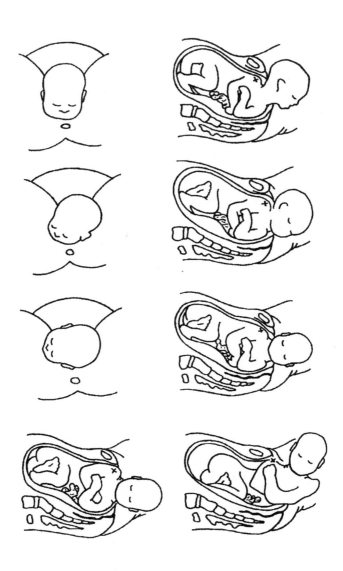

Section Two

A Look At The Anatomy

Section Two: The Anatomy And Physiology Of The Maternal Pelvis And The Foetal Head

"It's a bit like a jigsaw; when we're building the sky, the pieces may look the same, but there's only one space they will fit into without using force."

If we are to be able to understand how the birth process works, and why there are so many variations in the way each birthing pair manages it, we need to look again at the anatomy we learnt as students. It is surprising how little we are taught about the female pelvis. Even many of our models are deficient in lots of ways.

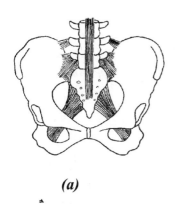

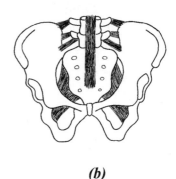

(a)

(b)

*Female Pelvis - Standing
Wider, lighter with shallow
pubic arch. Coccyx level with
or higher than symphasis*

*Male Pelvis - Standing
Strong and deep with
narrow pubic arch. Coccyx
lower than symphasis*

The female pelvis is structurally quite different to the male. Not only is it much lighter, it is more flexible, especially during pregnancy and birth. The sacrum measures the same, but it's curve is much more pronounced, meaning that the female coccyx is level with the middle, or sometimes even the top, of the symphasis, while in the male it is level with, or even lower than the lower border of the pubes. This is easily verified by inspecting lateral X-rays or scans.

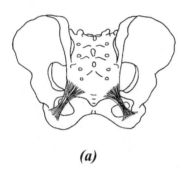

(a)

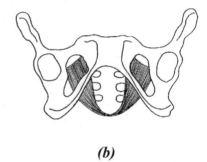

(b)

Female Pelvis - Standing Rear View. Note relationship between coccyx and pubes

Female Pelvis - Sitting Note how pelvic floor completely changes once coccyx is lower than pubes

Another point that becomes obvious, is the key role of the ischial tuberosities or more correctly, the way they relate to the spine and legs. By sitting on them and moving the body backwards and forwards, the way the front of the pelvis opens and closes is easily felt. It also shows why a baby finds becoming O P so simple!! As the spine moves backwards, the baby goes with it, and as he'd find facing backwards so close to the bony spine uncomfortable, he will turn to lie against it.

If we now stand up and repeat the exercise, we will feel how far the symphasis drops away from the spine. This is because as the legs straighten the angle between spine and pubes increases. During late pregnancy, as the lordosis (swayback) develops, this becomes even greater. The baby gets little support unless he turns to become O A. Any other position has him feeling as if he is lying on his face in a hammock, so he will happily settle with his back in the curve.

All this shows us why *deep* squatting is a " no-no".In societies where women squat during birth--only during second stage--people have squatted to urinate or defaecate since childhood. Thus, they squat *with their private parts facing the ground.* When westerners squat, they are unable to balance in this position, so assume a deep squat. This closes the pelvis, and *has the private parts facing the wall.* Instead of a wide- open doorway, there is a half- closed one. Even worse, if he is able to get his shoulders into the pelvis at all, the baby must go around the outside of the curve instead of across the short side.

Obviously then going to bed and reclining is also causing problems. We have all said at some time---"push him down and round the corner ". There shouldn't be a corner. If the mother is upright, with her legs lower than her body, the pelvis is open, the sacrum and coccyx are moved up and out and the outlet increases to 16cm.

When we look at the female pelvis, we see also that the distance between the ischial spines is much wider, and the sides straighter, making the bony outlet much bigger. As we noted above, the posterior wall has a much deeper curve, which is used by the baby when tucking in his head. Also, the arch of the symphasis is much wider and rounder.

The pelvis is wider from side to side at the top, and from front to back at the bottom, but the baby is wider (longer) from front to back at the top, and from side to side at the shoulders. Thus the easiest way out for the baby is, head down, facing backwards so that he can follow the pelvic curve. It's a bit like a jigsaw; when we're building the sky, the pieces may look the same, but there's only one space they will fit into without using force.

The Amazing Rhombus Of Michaelis.

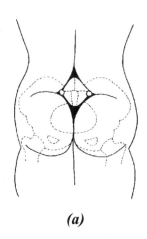

(a)

**Rhombus of Michaelis
Relationship to pelvis**

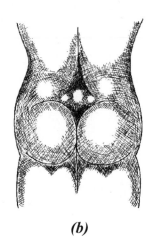

(b)

**Rhombus of Michaelis
Outside view of posterior**

This is the kite shaped area that includes the three lower lumbar vertebrae and the sacral prominence. As the sacrum is effectively fused, the whole posterior pelvic wall is involved.

We are never taught about the rhombus and its crucial role in second stage labour.

The action of the rhombus has obviously been unseen since women began to give birth with clothes on, and either in the lateral or supine position. As more mothers have given birth in upright and mobile postures, without wearing clothes, many midwives and support people have been privileged to see it rise in the maternal back as the baby began it's emergence. It appears to be controlled by a set of nerves approximating those affecting the male prostate gland. It was recognised by Andrea Robertson, that it was the area that in feminist literature is known as the G-Spot.

These are not the nerves of defaecation or deliberate pushing, but cause the "foetal ejection " reflex. They include in the voluntary system; the pelvic plexus of the inferior hypogastric nerve, and the clitoral nerve, and in the involuntary system the pelvic splanchnic nerve. Its action seems to be triggered in a normal birth by the back of the baby's neck pressing on these nerves as he begins to lift his head.

The rhombus moves quite differently from the so-called "nodding" action that we are taught. At the beginning of real physiological second stage labour, it moves backwards approx. 1-2cm and pushes the wings of the ilia outwards as it does so. This increases the outlet to around 16cm according to New Zealand obstetrician and midwifery tutor, Dr T.F. Corkill. (Deceased).

This knowledge was common among Jamaican midwives, who taught Sheila Kitzenger that "the baby will not be born until she opens her back". It is interesting that no-one felt inspired to enquire just what they meant.

Of course, just like women, pelvises are not identical. In fact, there are several major variations of them. We learn about the four pelvic shapes; gynaecoid, anthropoid, android, and platypeloid. These we will look at shortly, to see how they affect the ease with which the baby enters and passes through the pelvis.

During the last few weeks of pregnancy, the lordosis of pregnancy should be established, increasing the useable space between the sacral prominence and pubes. The ligaments should have softened; giving the characteristic "duck waddle" that indicates a straightforward Occipito-anterior labour and birth. The uterus will have assumed its final position tilted to the maternal right and turned slightly to the left at its base--(the right obliquity and dextrorotation of the textbooks) The tissues of the mother's vagina and pelvic floor become soft and stretchy.

All these changes are brought about by hormonal stimulation, as the baby prepares to move from his once comfortable home to the world. If he fails to assume the optimal position of Left occipito-anterior as a first, or Right occipito- anterior as an alternative for a later one, he does not give the necessary signals strongly enough to encourage his mother's birth passage tissues to relax and let him emerge.

The tables on the following page explain the measurements of the maternal pelvis and the foetal head in more detail.

MEASUREMENTS OF THE PELVIS

Normally

	Transverse	Oblique	Ant.Post
Brim	13	12	11
Cavity	12	12	12
Outlet	11	12	13

Second stage - after rhombus opens

	Transverse	Oblique	Ant.Post
Brim	15	14	13
Cavity	14	14	14
Outlet	13	14	15

MEASUREMENTS OF FOETAL HEAD

	Diameters	Circumference
OA	9.5 x 9.5 cm	27.5 cm
OP	11.5 x 9.5 cm	35.5 cm

The Foetal Skull

The foetal skull is also something we don't learn enough about. The dangers of excessive moulding are taught, but that rarely happens if the baby is tucked up properly.

There is no discussion of the difference between the folding along sutures to decrease the head diameter, and the moulding or change of shape of the parietals that occurs when some part other than the occiput presents. There is a real need to understand these bones in order to assess the effects on the baby. In folding there should be no effect on the contents of the skull, while in moulding, the meninges, blood vessels, nerves, lymphatics as well as the ventricles containing the cerebro-spinal fluid, are liable to stretching and / or distortion. The dreaded tentorial tear is the extreme outcome of serious moulding

A baby in an Occipito-posterior (O P) position, subjected to close, strong contractions, and forced into the lower segment rather than onto the cervix, may develop some or all of the following:

- Compression of bones of cervical spine between skull and shoulders.

- A distorted occiput---remember, it's in four moveable pieces---which may press on or stretch the vagus nerve, and the effects eventually be seen on the monitor tracing as "foetal distress".

- Development of the large caput--Often with the bony skull still above the spines, or even on odd occasions the brim.

- Developing later: Difficulty with feeding--the hypoglossal nerve is pinched, and he is unable to bring his tongue down from the roof of his mouth. Normal handling and flexing of his body will often correct this, but an osteopath will fix it at once. All that is needed is to *carefully* lift his head forward, away from his shoulders, and the instant relaxation tells you that his neck is free.

- Glue ear or chronic otitis media. The mastoid process is undeveloped at birth, and it is simple for the movement of the basal skull bones to bend the eustachian tube between throat and inner ear. This prevents proper drainage of any secretions, and so chronic infection is likely.

- Squints or shortsightedness - the orbit has eight small bones forming its bony shape. Each has one or more tiny muscle attached to it. If these are moved even a hairsbreadth, the eye is not held at its proper angle.

*** See Diagrams Over Page**

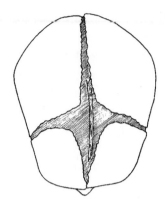

Top of skull

Note membraneous areas

Foetal skull - side view
Note: large membraneous
area below parietals and in
front of occiput.

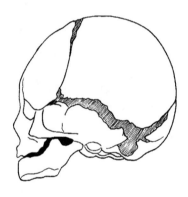

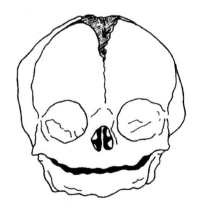

Foetal head - front view

Note many small bones in orbits
(eye sockets) and behind nose.

The only skull bones that have assumed their final shape at birth are the frontals and parietals. All the others are in several pieces - though enclosed in the same "case" and some haven't even started to grow. We worry about the vault of his skull, but that is the most difficult part to damage. The base of his head may be grown from cartilage, but it is still soft, and the bones are a lot like pieces of playing card enclosed in two layers of clingfilm.

His head is especially designed so that if, once again, he is in the best position for birth, he is able to tuck it right back into the curve of his mother's sacrum. Then, if he needs more room, he can fold the bones of his vault. The occiput and frontal bones pass under the parietals and the leading one of those over the other. Thus, there is no strain or tension on any part of his head.

He is safe enough as a left sacrum anterior breech also, as long as his mother stays on her feet or knees, and he is able to turn his head in the right direction. He gets into trouble if his mother lies down and he is unable to help himself.

It is the baby in the Occipito- posterior position who has the problems. Thus with each contraction, his neck and the base of his head must take all the pressure. This is probably well in front of the cervix, on the lower uterine segment, which provides far more resistance. Contractions augmented by syntocinon can cause much greater distortion.

Even if he is finally " rescued " by operative procedures, his skull has no mechanism to allow the displaced sections of bone to return to their proper place. If he is lucky, he will be tucked up beside his mother and allowed to rest --just as if he had concussion; which is probably exactly what he has!

Maybe the old idea of holding newborns upside down by the feet had its advantages, as the relatively heavy head would have pulled the neck and skull base free!

This brief outline should already have us thinking about ways to protect the baby's head from such stress. Many of his problems can be helped after birth by osteopathy (cranio--sacral) or gentle chiropractic treatment, but it would be much better if we could prevent the damage occurring in the first place! *Prevention is better than cure!*

As we look at each pelvic type, and each foetal presentation, we will concentrate on non-invasive ways to help.

Variations In Pelvic Shape, And How They Affect The Birth Process

Most women today are well shaped. There are no longer pelvises deformed by rickets, tuberculosis and osteomyelitis, as there were when I first began work. If birth again becomes a normal female life event, regarded as part of the community continuum, (No, I'm not advocating babies being born in public!) where the community values its mothers, we midwives will be the facilitators. To do this we must understand just how the shape of the maternal pelvis affects the ease with which the baby enters the pelvis, as well as the course of labour. Once we have learnt to watch the way mothers walk and stand, we begin to realise that the differences can be seen quite clearly. Watching girl children run is even more instructive. The ones with " good " pelvises look awkward as they swing their legs around their pelvis. The android types run tidily like boys.

An American doctor, Howard C. Molloy M.D. M.Sc. in 1951 published a comprehensive clinical and roentgenological evaluation of the pelvis (published by W B. Saunders Company.) This is very helpful if allowance is made for the fact that many of the X-rays on which the conclusions are based were taken with women in sitting or reclining positions.

Types of Pelvis

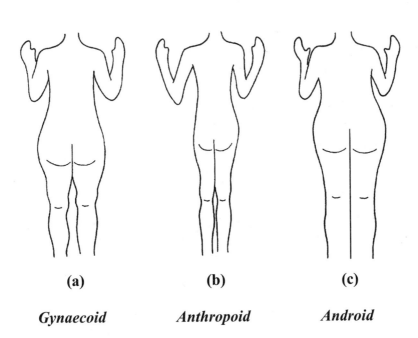

(a)	(b)	(c)
Gynaecoid	*Anthropoid*	*Android*

The Three Main Female Figure Types

(a) The Gynaecoid

Among western women the most common is the gynaecoid pelvis, which is the easiest for babies to enter at the correct angle. It is found in around 50% of women, and is recognisable externally once its appearance is understood. The woman appears to have shoulders slightly narrower than her hips. She will also have a slim waist. Her hips are broad and well rounded, but her lower legs tend to be quite slim. If she runs, she must swing her legs outwards round the base of her pelvis. This can be seen in quite young girls. This is the woman who looks dreadful in trousers, too round, and too much bottom.

Even a baby coming to labour as an O P will be able to rotate into O A if his mother is mobile---the open front of the pelvis, and the shape of the symphasis make things easier. Passing the "spines" is simple, because there is plenty of space behind the symphasis for the widest part of his head, and this baby needs no help to emerge.

(b) The Anthropoid

This occurs in about 24% of women and its main effect is to increase the likelihood of the baby assuming the O P (occipito posterior position). This woman has wide shoulders and narrow hips, and a slightly thicker waist than a gynaecoid type. She is likely to be tall and slender, with "good " legs---that is her inner thighs, knees, calves and ankles touch with open spaces between them.

The baby will often enter the pelvis in the oblique diameter, as the inlet shape is deeper from front to back than in the gynaecoid type. As long as the mother is mobile during labour, things may take a little longer than in an O A birth. The pelvis has rather straight sides so the distance between the spines is often more easily negotiated. There is as usual with O.P.s, noticeably more discomfort for the mother, so encouraging the baby to become O A before labour is still important. The baby in this type of pelvis is the one who finds pelvic floor rotation relatively simple.

(c) The Android

The android pelvis occurs in a little over 20% of western women. It is found in women who look quite "Square " from behind. Their legs are usually solid from hips to ankles, sometimes ending abruptly in small feet. These women walk without having to move their legs round their pelvis, but may walk on the inner aspect of their feet instead of the outer---they have legs that touch all the way down, so are more likely to suffer from chafing of the thighs.

This type of pelvis causes little difficulty at the brim. There may well be an acute angle at the symphasis, meaning that the baby will be unable to use a lot of the anterior space. As its name implies, it is a masculine type pelvis---its funnel shape continuing to the outlet. Here the labour that has been going well slows down. This mother will probably have to push her baby out. She will also need to focus on ways to increase her internal pelvic diameters. Changing from upright to side-lying, and sometimes even flat on her back for a couple of contractions, to avoid the forceps "help ". Stair walking is ideal, but hardly likely to appeal during second stage. The increase in outlet diameter from movement of the rhombus of Michaelis is very important for this birthing pair.

(d) The Platypeloid

This is not common, but very easily recognised. If someone says, "she looks good in trousers"- beware! She will have a very wide lateral brim diameter, but a short anterior -posterior one. She will also have a fairly flat sacral curve. In some cases the symphasis is much thicker than normal --- even feeling on vaginal examination like the underside of a shelf. If in doubt, ask her to turn side on, and the narrow anterior -posterior pelvis is obvious. This mother will usually have an O P baby, who causes great discomfort as he tries to turn to the L O A. It is very difficult for him to enter the pelvis,-- Right-occipito-posterior (R O P), or right-occipito-lateral (R O L) so he must try to turn right across his mother's symphasis. This is extremely painful -entering pains can be even more painful than labour. They are also erratic, sometimes lasting up to 10 - 20 (ten to twenty) minutes. They may also continue for several hours, reducing the mother to tears. Many mothers lift the whole uterus off the pubes to reduce the discomfort, so preventing the baby's efforts succeeding. His head must be absolutely lateral if he is to have any chance of entering the maternal pelvis. Fortunately, once he's in he's as good as born, as there is normally plenty of space between the "spines" and a short straight sacrum giving a good outlet.

These mothers and those with android pelvises are the women who had most of the terribly difficult births that " Old wives' tales " dwell on.

In most cases, the pelvis will be a modification or combination of types, though one will predominate. Learning to recognise them pays good dividends. The mothers who are likely to have problems can have extra information about ways to improve their baby's birth. The ones with real difficulties will get help earlier---watchful expectancy won't get an R O P into a platypeloid pelvis, but left side sleeping added to regular use of forward leaning postures does. A baby in an android pelvis needs more help than one in a gynaecoid one.

Elizabeth's Story

Elizabeth is waiting for her first baby to engage. She is 37weeks pregnant, and her family are telling her that she'll have an easy time because she has "child-bearing" hips. Her midwife, the mother of two herself feels doubtful. She has a platypeloid pelvis, and thinks that Elizabeth looks a lot like her. She talks to Elizabeth's mother, and hears that she and one of her sisters, spent several days in labour after their "waters" broke. The midwife decides to explain about the need for interaction between mother and unborn, if the same thing is not to recur.

Fortunately Elizabeth's husband grasps the importance of the relationship of the baby's head and its mother's pelvis if things are to go well. He encourages efforts to persuade the baby to move---forward leaning and left side resting and sleeping especially. It was very hard to keep trying, as the baby was R.O.L. and getting over to the left was extremely painful. The best relief came from being on all fours and lifting the whole abdomen towards Elizabeth's ribs. It took around ten days before things settled to a good foetal position.

At the same time, Elizabeth's cousin Joy, who was due to have her baby 3 weeks before Elizabeth, and who had no advice about helping her baby, had Spontaneous Rupture of Membranes with her baby still above the brim.

She had no contractions after 12 hours, so P.G.s were inserted. Joy was confined to bed, propped up with pillows, and very unhappy with the pain of baby's head moving. Still nothing-after 24 hours from S.R.M.-cervix 1.5cm long, tightly closed and very posterior. A syntocinon infusion, plus an epidural for pain relief was tried, but the baby was still high after 6 hours. A caesarian section for disproportion was done to end the torment for mother and especially the baby.

Maybe if Joy had been up and about once a V.E. had confirmed that there was no cord presenting, things may have progressed. However a full term baby trying to enter a platypeloid pelvis usually takes up to four days, with long "Braxton Hicks" shaped contractions. It is much easier for a baby to enter at the usual 37-38 weeks, but for this to happen, the mother and her support people must accept the idea of maternal-- foetal interaction. As around 2-3% of women have some degree of this A P narrowing, there is a real need for midwifery help.

Even when there is early S. R. M. there is no damage to the baby's head as long as he remains above the brim. So apart from the danger of infection- which is slight if the mother remains at home and V.E.s are avoided, - it is possible to wait for labour to start. However, there would be very few mothers who wanted to wait, as this situation is the one of those on which the many of the horror stories of the past are based.

Effects of the Foetal Head Shape on Labour

The way the shape of a baby's head influences the course of labour is seldom considered. However the baby with a nicely shaped head will have a much easier time, both with entering the maternal pelvis, and leaving the maternal body.

A baby with either a really round or almost square head has nothing to lead with, so the lower uterine segment is unable to mould it effectively. How often does a small 3000gram (approximately) sized baby end up needing ventouse, forceps or even caesarian section to be born? Some of them are perfectly shaped after a long tedious labour ---as if they'd been born by elective section, and never been in the pelvis.

There will be families within a given group who always have problems. Some babies have bi-parietal diameters up to 1cm greater than average, so if they are trying to enter a normal sized pelvis they must do so early, while their skull bones are soft. These babies may also have heads that are flat on top, thus reducing the chances of folding along the sutures.

There is really no way open to midwifery to measure the shape of an unborn's head, so we must rely on family histories. Doctors may order an ultra-sound scan, so if one is available the technician may be able to assess the head shape. Where midwives do their own scans, a great opportunity is to be had. There are very few situations where the baby is unable to enter the pelvic brim once appropriate action is taken.

In really old Greek society the midwives chose who would partner whom. After all they were the ones expected to deal with the results. Sometimes it looks like a good idea for today too.

A baby with the classic measurements of bi-parietals 9.5cm, bi-temporals of 8.5cm, and occipito-frontal of 11.5cm will make the best use of all the available space. The commonest difference seems to be in the bi-temporal, which may well be the same as the bi-parietal, giving the "sweet" round head and face. The "square" head often has a shortened occipito-frontal as well, which also means there is nothing for the uterus to mould.

The Shape of the Neck

Another aspect that never seems to be mentioned is the shape of the baby's neck. O.A. s as we all know, have fat folds at the back of their necks. This enables them to tuck their chins right down level with their breastbones, and fit up under the maternal sacrum facing upwards. This is why, when the mother is fully dilated and about to be told " you can push now" (such arrogance, she's not ready) the foetal heart is heard behind the symphasis, but the head is still 3cm or more away from the outlet.

This flexion is important, as the baby presenting in any other position, including breech has less neck rolls, and thus much less flexibility throughout his life. That is, the meninges surrounding his brain and spinal cord are tight and such things as "forward rolls" or gymnastic moves are likely to be difficult and may even be painful.

Once we start looking at the wider picture of anatomical relationships between mother and baby we find it increasingly simple to find ways to make life easier for everyone involved in the birth process. As we learn ways to encourage the babies to move their backs to their mother's left sides, from where they can easily become L O L--A we will find our workload dramatically reduced. Postmaturity becomes much less common, and thus the need for inductions with their propensity for setting off the well known "cascade of intervention". The baby's skull bones will still be quite soft and able to fold along the sutures. We do need to look at the way the baby's head shape is changed during the process of birth. The O.A who engages early is both folded and moulded, while the one who engages late, but emerges quickly may be simply folded along the sutures.

The O.P is more moulded than folded, as his parietal bones must become more elongated if he is to fit. It is hard for 11.5cm to fit through a 10cm dilated cervix!

We rarely stop to consider the effects on the interior of baby's head from excessive moulding. The extreme of tentorial tear we are well aware of, but there must also be stretching of the meninges where any marked degree of moulding occurs.

Have we thought that maybe, just maybe, foetal distress is caused in part by the trapping of the vagus nerve as it passes through the occiput? After all, the fusion of the four parts into one bone happens after birth. There are many other places where movement between bones, or parts of bones, may happen, and there appears to be no mechanism to correct this. This movement rarely occurs when the baby is O.A as he flexes his head onto his chest, thus removing any resistance. In any other position, the full force of contractions enters the base of his skull and must have some result. It is not often that an O.A baby needs "rescuing" unless he is in an android pelvis, and his mother is confined to bed.

If we are aware that many babies in a family have had difficult births, and that they have awkwardly shaped heads, we can talk with the mother at around 34 weeks gestation, about ways to get her baby into the best possible position while it is still easy. Being faced with this situation once labour is well established is a challenge that is not always possible to overcome.

Let Birth Be Born Again!

Section Three

Antenatal Care

Section Three: Antenatal Care

"Good antenatal information and education is the key to making a baby's entry into this world a simpler and safer process."

The exciting thing for midwifery is that there is a great deal that can be done to avoid O P presentations happening.

When we look at the O A baby, we see that he is commonly in the multigravida's abdomen, with its apple shaped uterus and less firm muscles. It is quite easy for this baby to rotate, as long as his mother avoids resting in reclining positions. She tends to do a lot of forward leaning, picking up after the toddler.

Most of us are familiar with the mother almost "caught short" by number two after a long tedious first birth. It's always amazed me that any of us are brave enough to try again!!

We know that a first baby has really only two options in a vertex presentation. L O A if he's lucky, or his mother knows what he needs and helps him get it, or R O P which is the direct opposite angle.

Left occipito posterior (L O P) is an extremely rare choice and it's not hard to see why. The maternal stomach and colon are in the way, and the lean to the right at the top of the uterus would make it a very uncomfortable place to be. Babies aren't silly! Like the rest of us they take the easiest route they can.

R O A is also difficult for first babies for similar reasons. The lower segment, with its twist to the left, that hasn't been stretched by a labour and foetal descent, combined with the lean to the right at the top and the obstructions on the maternal left make it difficult. The tight abdominal muscles also make a difference. Since aerobics and serious exercises became popular, more multip's babies are having problems.

Mothers with babies in the occipito-posterior position have a miserable late pregnancy and birth. They look very neat and tidy and are generally praised as "carrying so well".

Unfortunately, it is because the baby is lying high in the maternal abdomen with his head straight. He will be on her right side, with his back in the curve between her spine and hip. His head will normally be in the oblique R O P, moving to the transverse---R O L as he attempts to enter the pelvis.

As the maternal sacrum projects well out over the pelvic brim (most of these mothers have very little lordosis) he is unable to bend his neck far enough to begin to engage. Braxton Hicks contractions have no effect on his efforts to change position. He needs to be able to bring his bottom well out into his mother's abdomen to find enough room, and this will not happen until real labour contractions change the uterine shape.

Unborn babies have very short necks, but should have several very fat folds at the back that normally allow them to bring their chins down on their chests. O.P. s do not develop these properly, so can bend only as far as an adult can, and then not until they pass the "spines" and flex against the pelvic floor. Post maturity is a common feature of O.P presentations.

How To Help

The first thing is to believe that you can make a difference, even if you work in a busy antenatal clinic.

Many areas are setting up continuity of care schemes, and these are just what is needed (total one-to-one care will be too hard to keep up, but there are many ways to create small groups caring for all the women in a given area and for the whole pregnancy)

Giving the antenatal, intra-partum and postnatal care is the ideal, but even if only the clinic is involved a lot can be done. Pregnant women love the company of other pregnant women, so if the clinic did nothing more than encourage networks from geographical areas it would still be valuable. *However, once the clinic staff decide to make increasing the number of normal presentations a priority, amazing things can happen.*

At each visit the mother is asked to describe what her baby has been doing in the last few days. Listen to her.

At first, many will be too shy and wonder what it's for. If the midwife tells the mother why she listens to the baby's heartbeat in a particular place, the mother is likely to say such things as;

- "I felt him poking his knees out last night "
- "We could feel him stretching his arms and legs today".
- "He had the hiccups all last night "
- "There's this great big bulge under my ribs " and
- "I can feel him nodding his head "---this tells you straight away that he's currently a breech.

Once that trust is established it is time to start talking about how to make things easier for themselves during the birth. The idea that any vertex position will do is a fallacy. Very few babies turn in early labour, especially if they are first ones. So explain that the baby needs to lie on her left side with his back to her front, and head down by approximately weeks 34 -36.

Making Birth Easier And Simpler For All

The Midwife's Role

The midwife is the 'keeper' of the knowledge the mother needs if she is to work with, instead of against her baby's efforts. Communicating this knowledge effectively is vitally important. Antenatal information and education are the key to making a baby's entry to this world a simpler safer process. We know which ones have the easy trip, so how do we convince more of them to do it that way?

We need to accept that babies know what they must do. Any mother will be able to describe the efforts her baby made to line itself up properly. Unfortunately, very few find the efforts comfortable, so instead of helping most mothers hinder .The horrid rubbing of the baby's head on the inside of the maternal symphasis is never really forgotten. We are often so thoughtless as to tell the induced mother experiencing this pain that it is "only the baby's head moving" - as if she didn't already know that!!

When it happens before labour, most women lie down on their backs, in itself a giant mistake, and then lift the base of their abdomen upwards. This certainly stops the pain, but it also means that eventually the baby gives up trying and falls back into the O P position.

If the mother, and equally as important her support people, have been shown with a doll and model pelvis just what is needed, then a leaning forward position makes sense. The idea is to make sure that the baby is uncomfortable in any but the right position. By leaning forward, the mother removes the support her abdominal muscles have been giving, and the baby feels as if he is trying to lie on his face in a hammock. This isn't nice, so he quickly starts to turn. Whether it is just leaning against the kitchen bench, or over a beanbag, or adopting a hands and knees stance, the weight of the baby is taken off the symphasis and he has room to rotate without resistance. Of course he has to be awake and ready to move before it's any use trying to move him. Well meaning family, and often, professional caregivers, advise mothers to rest, without the qualification that it must be in a side-lying attitude.

A Bad Position for mum and baby

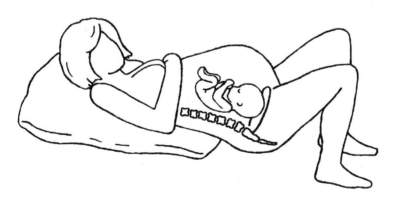

Reclining causes more problems than it solves

The old-fashioned 'chaise-longue' used by Victorian upper classes was the right idea. Modern lounge furniture is especially bad for mothers in the last weeks of pregnancy. Their bottoms are kept lower than their knees, and their abdomens higher than their spines. The puffy legs may need raising, but reclining causes more problems than it solves.

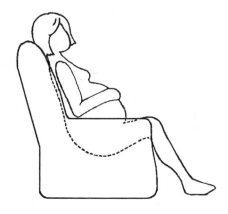

Modern Lounge Furniture is especially bad for mothers in the last weeks of pregnancy.

Another 'no -no' is deep squatting. Fortunately very few women find it possible in late pregnancy. It brings the spine and symphasis too close together and makes the upright baby even more so. The angle between spine and pubes must be kept as wide as possible

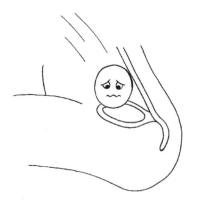

Squatting - Western women bring their spine forward and bottom down, closing the inlet and tightening the pelvic floor.

Postures that keep women upright, kneeling or leaning forward, or properly designed maternity stools are the answer. The stools have wide seats and knee rests that enable the mother to rotate her hips outwards, thus also relieving the backache of late pregnancy. A side benefit is that the "bulge" fits under the table, and the mother can sit closer to her food thus helping to keep her clothes clean!

They also allow the baby to move until his back is between his mother's left hip and umbilicus. From here it is easy for him to slip his posterior parietal into the curve of the sacrum, rest against the inner aspect of the pubes, and begin the turn to L O A. A firm wedge shaped cushion can also be used to tip the pelvis forward. From there, a spontaneous, on-time labour and birth can be expected. *The mother must realise that if when sitting she can cross her legs, her bottom is too low.*

If the baby is really unco-operative, " tummy down " resting with lots of supporting pillows under head and legs, as well as between bosom and bulge will help. Just like a hammock, the only comfortable lie for baby is L O A. Swimming, using a relaxed overarm movement, walking, or yoga type exercises are really good for pregnant women. All these change the internal angles between spine and pelvis and offer the baby a chance to turn. *Mobility and movement in response to the baby's efforts is the key.*

There should always be a model pelvis and a decent sized doll in every midwife's bag, antenatal clinic and *delivery suite.

(Who called it delivery by the way? Doesn't the word say a lot about our attitudes and us? A baby in the correct position, being helped by its mother doesn't need to be 'delivered'. In fact it's a contradiction in terms. A baby is either born or delivered. The terms are not interchangeable!)

The midwife's responsibility is to reassure the mother that her efforts to co-operate with her baby will be fruitful.

Great patience will be needed if the baby is in an O.P position, but almost all babies will turn if the mother perseveres. Mothers can cope with the discomfort, or sometimes-even real pain of the baby rubbing against the inside of the pubes, if they understand the reward for persevering.

If her partner is included in discussions of the baby's needs, it is usually found that he understands the engineering aspects more easily, and can see the importance of protecting the baby's head while it is being born.

Dads are great allies and once they see what we mean, will often be more aware of the baby's position.

Properly Designed Maternity Stools Are The Answer

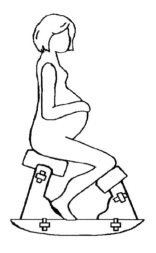

<u>*Useful Upright And Forward Leaning Postures*</u>

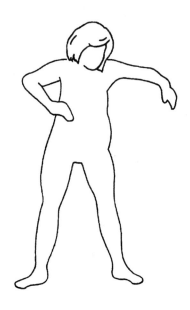

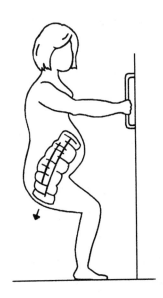

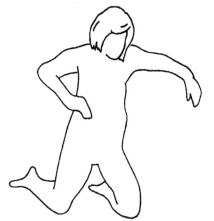

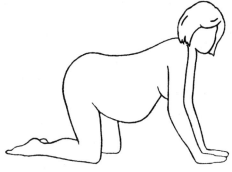

Key points - What Mothers Need To Know

- That birth is a co-operative action between mother and baby.

- That babies try very hard to assume the best position for birth.

- That she must if possible keep her knees lower than her bottom.

- That when resting, she should lie on her left side with her legs level with her body.

- That her baby's efforts to turn across her pubes will be between uncomfortable and painful.

- That she can minimise this by adopting forward leaning postures while her baby is moving.

- That there is no point in trying to move her baby when he is sleeping. Wait till he wakes.

- That when her abdomen sags, and her back aches, it is better to wear a girdle than to tuck her tail under. Expect some lordosis.

- That once her baby is in the best position, the only small lump she will feel, is far round between her hip bone and ribs.

- That a baby in the best position gives good signals to his mothers body to prepare to let him out easily for both of them. Remaining upright and mobile will aid labour.

- That this baby is likely to be born on time, and proceed just as the books tell us.

- That he will come out with a minimum of effort, in as short a time as possible, and arrive peaceful, unstressed and ready to get on with life.

- That chemical pain relief is not likely to be needed, as the mother's body will respond to her baby's signals, and she will cope magnificently.

Teach the Concept of Available Space

Passage and passenger remain the same size, but by manoeuvring and changing their inter-relationship, one may pass through the other.

Below a floating ball in a bottle of liquid represents the baby and the pelvis. Notice how the **available space** (seen by the horizontal line) can be altered to give the baby more room to manoeuvre.

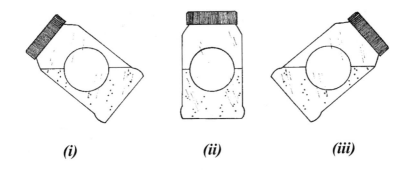

(i)   *(ii)*   *(iii)*

How Tilting the Pelvis Changes the Available Space

(i)   Lean left - raise right leg - for baby R. O. L -P not engaged by 38 weeks. Also for failure to descend in 2nd stage (right shoulder on brim)

(ii)   Upright - Minimal moving room

(iii)   Lean right - raise left leg - for L. O. A trying to rotate at the brim. Also if shoulders are not transverse at 2nd stage.

Effects of a Change of Posture on the Available Space

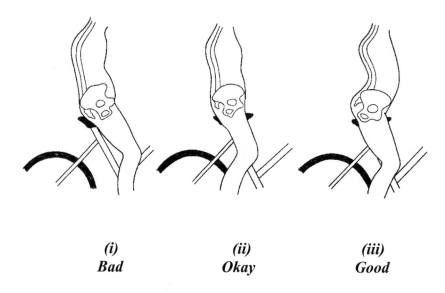

(i)	*(ii)*	*(iii)*
Bad	*Okay*	*Good*

How Small Body Movements Alter the Space at the Brim and Outlet

(i)   Back rounded, weight behind tuberosities - result - Flat brim and closed outlet.

(ii)   Back straight, well balanced - result - Inlet open.

(iii)   Back arched - result - Inlet and outlet wide open. Plenty of space.

Antenatal Classes.

If midwives believe in normal birth and women's ability to achieve it, they will see that becoming seriously involved in antenatal education is a priority. It provides access to pregnant women and equally as important their support people. The times optimal foetal positioning fails are almost always where the partner laughs at the idea. Pregnant women are very sensitive to words and attitudes. Small classes mean that we have to keep on repeating ourselves, but much of what is in current classes could be left out, or reduced to a minimum. If most mothers are going to achieve the normal O A, there is no need for in-depth talk of epidurals and interventions. Once they are relegated to their proper place as emergency procedures, we will again be able to practise as midwives, rather than obstetric nurses.

Achieving the optimal position for birth is possible for at least 85 percent of babies, and if we consider only the vertex presentations there is no reason why 95 percent of them can't manage it.

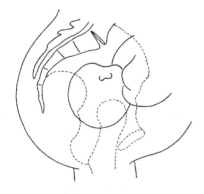

Engaged L.O.A

Note the amount of space around the head

Special exercises would not be needed if we reverted to our "old-fashioned" lifestyles, where women spent hours over a washtub, scrubbing floors and doorsteps and growing the family food. However, that's a bit drastic, so we'll have to find other ways to help.

Most of today's classes focus on socialising mothers and support people to accept the care given by whichever unit provides it. Unfortunately, protocols tend to vary according to the wishes of the most senior practitioner, and many have no research basis. "Prevention rather than cure " is seldom the primary objective.

Couples who question practises are seen as a threat, rather than a challenge. It does us good to look at our actions, and see which ones are just habits, good or bad, and which ones really make a difference to outcomes.

Fragmented care often means that mothers are given hopes that the birth they want will be supported by the staff in " Delivery Suite " who are probably frantically busy, trying to care for several women at once and quite unable to spend the extra time needed to find non-invasive ways to help. The fact that it saves time as the labour progresses is overruled by the immediate demands of the unit.

All this means that the birthing family needs to be taught how to help themselves. Back-rubbing techniques, perineal massage, you name it, most of these things actually get in the way of the mother developing her own labour rhythm and entering into the detached endorphin state. The use of water tubs, or birth pools may reduce the amount of pain, but unless the mother is able to assume a forward leaning position, these will do nothing to shorten the labour.
Breathing exercises are yet another "survival" technique.

Accurate information about her baby's position, and stage of labour that she has reached is vital so that she can cooperate effectively.

During Classes

During classes, couples can be taught how to recognise many signs for themselves. This will mean fewer mothers coming to hospital far too early, being put onto an antenatal floor and induced in the morning. All mothers and support people should understand that a straightforward labour is only possible if the baby is L O A, and how to recognise this.

- The mother's abdomen will be bulky and well out in front.
- Her umbilicus will protrude.
- Her labia and pelvic floor will feel warm and bulky and often most uncomfortable when she sits.
- A tiny lump will poke out right round on her right side between hip and ribs as her baby stretches a leg.
- Sleeping should be easier as long as she lies on her left side, though she may feel that she needs a skinny cushion under the "bulge".
- She will have a duck-waddle way of walking.
- Her breasts may well be secreting colostrum during the last few days.

During the preparation stage, if the baby is still not settled properly into the pelvis, the following will probably happen:

- The baby's efforts to turn will trigger "sets" of contractions, that will often be regular at 5 minutes, but last between 30 and 60 seconds. These may continue for several hours, but are not effacing or dilating the cervix.

What Will Help

The contractions will stop if the mother takes a warm bath, or a relaxing massage. They also stop when the baby gets tired of trying. This is not desirable, so if the mother wants to help her baby, then she should assume any tummy down posture she can. These include leaning over a beanbag; sitting backwards on a kitchen chair with a cushion under her bottom; practising "cat arches " of her back while on hands and knees on the floor; lying face down on the bed with pillows under head and legs and between bosoms and bulge. This is when all her mother's spare pillows come in handy!

Should the mother be in a car, she should stop (somewhere safe) and get out to lean on the car, with her tummy relaxed. However it's done, the key is to get the abdomen low and relaxed, so that the baby literally topples into it. This is where a supportive partner is so important. The mother becomes demoralised if she feels that she is alone in her efforts.

Birth Day

Expectant parents need to know how women behave during labour. The heightened sense of excitement of early labour. The talkative phase as things settle into a rhythm, then the more abstracted state, as contractions become established.

Now the abdomen is changing shape with each one, and the mother's eyes cease to focus clearly. There is no need to time contractions. Once they are strong enough to have her catching her breath and grasping a support, it is time to prepare. First babies don't fall out in bathrooms very often!!

The Changing Shape of the Abdomen between Contractions

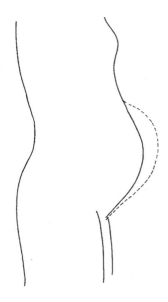

Note change in body shape.

Full line - between contractions

Dotted line - during contractions

These changes occur only when real labour begins. During a "working" contraction the sides of the uterus straighten, the top flattens and the uterus tilts forward. If in bed the uterus "rears" up.

If the mother remains upright and mobile this type of labour should, for first babies, last between 4 and 8 hours and for subsequent babies around 2 hours.

Parents should also learn about the less straightforward births, so that they can be prepared.

Understanding Why And When Her Baby Needs Help

By 36/40 weeks of pregnancy, the baby should be getting settled, ready for birth. Before then, there is less baby than bath water, or liquor, so the baby is free to change his position as often as he likes. Thus, although his mother has been learning how to help him, it has not always been successful. Now, things are different. The uterus has assumed its tilt to the right at the top, and its twist to the left at its base --that is, the right obliquity and dextro-rotation of the textbooks. Now for primigravida the right side is slightly shorter than the left, so there is more room for his back between mother's left hip and umbilicus.

He needs to be properly positioned by 38 weeks, as after this there is less liquor, and not much moving room. If he isn't settled, then serious efforts must be made to encourage him, by ensuring that he is uncomfortable facing forwards. Mother must keep her knees well down----no reclining to rest, as this makes a posterior position the most comfortable. All the tummy down postures must be persevered with, and if necessary, and if the idea is acceptable to the mother, now is the time for such things as homoeopathy, acupuncture, acupressure, etc. to be used. There are many practitioners specialising in care of the pregnant couple to consult.

Section Four

Some Success Stories

Section Four: Some Success Stories!

" Result - a very happy family, able to say confidently, ' We did it ourselves! ' "

Ante-Natal Rotation - Primigravida

Primigravida babies need to become settled earlier than multigravida's. This is because an entering head has not stretched the base of the uterus, so it is a pear shape. Also the cervix tends to be more posterior.

The mother's abdominal muscles are usually really tight by 36 / 38 weeks of pregnancy, making palpation of the baby difficult. If the mother is asked to focus on what her baby is doing, and a sonic aid or other portable ultrasound device follows the foetal heart sounds till the valves can be heard opening and closing, there is no point in deep palpation. In time, it will become irrelevant as a means of ascertaining the baby's position.

Carol's Story (1)

Carol was at clinic for her 36 weeks check. Her baby was still very active, turning from one side to the other several times a day. He could be seen to push his arms and legs forward, making "bumps" at the front of her abdomen. The feel of his head rubbing against her pubic bone and bladder was most unpleasant. When she rested, feet up on the couch, things felt worse. At these times she was inclined to lift her whole abdomen upward to stop the discomfort.

A scan confirmed that the baby's placenta was on the upper, back uterine wall, so the baby should be facing it. Why wasn't he? Probably because Carol did not understand the importance of forward leaning postures. Her baby was more comfortable in the O P erect position when Carol had her bottom lower than her knees or rested with her back lower than her abdomen.

Carol's midwife told her about the reasons for keeping her knees lower. At home, a special "maternity comfort rocker" will relieve backache, and provide a wide seat and knee rest. *She learns that a pregnant woman must be able to rotate her knees outward.* Also that resting for puffy legs should be done lying on her left side. This is important, as her baby will tip forward, with his head in the direct transverse, and be able to start entering her pelvis. If they are both on the right side--that is, baby has his back on her right, and she is lying on that side, rotation to L O A will be difficult as well as painful. He can't easily turn uphill. She was also shown, with doll and pelvis, why a baby who engages right-occipito-lateral is set for problems.

Carol and her partner took the advice seriously and Carol included lying over a beanbag to read, her book on the floor, and to watch television.

She found resisting people's efforts to persuade her to recline to rest the most difficult to deal with, so her partner's help was essential. Their midwife provided extra support over the phone when things got too hard.

At her 38 weeks check, Carol's midwife listened to baby's heartbeat on her left side, and assured her that as long as baby stayed where he was, labour would start close to the expected date and that her plan for an active, unmedicated birth would be realistic.

Carol's labour started at 40 weeks and 2 days. It progressed to a spontaneous vaginal birth, with Carol kneeling over a beanbag. No need for any pushing efforts. Baby's head appeared as Carol arched her back and thrust her pubis forward. Seconds later rotation was complete; the posterior shoulder emerged, then the anterior, followed by the rest of the body. Carol sat back on her heels and looked at her newborn. Ten minutes later the placenta was born, as baby suckled strongly at Mum's breast. Total time---4 hours and 20 minutes. No tear, no episiotomy. Result - a very happy family, able to say confidently "We did it ourselves!".

The midwife's role

Most of the important midwifery input was given during the antenatal checks and classes. Carol needed help to put the teaching into practice, as her family tried to have her rest reclining with her feet up, and found these "new ideas" hard to grasp at first. Her mother did eventually realise that she had assumed most of the recommended positions during her daily chores when her own family was arriving.

After the mandatory initial vital signs check and recording, there was little input needed. Checking the baby's heart beat at intervals, and providing a protective environment, where Carol felt able to follow her instincts, was all that was required. Watching and listening, reminding Carol to keep up her fluids and visit the toilet was the rest.

The baby birthing itself unaided was a new experience for this midwife. Happily she was fortunate enough to find a senior midwife who felt safe trusting women and their instincts, with whom she could discuss the event openly.

Bev's Story (2)

Bev was over 40 weeks pregnant with her first baby, when she and her partner came to see the midwife one morning. Her baby was a direct O P, well above the brim. His legs and arms could be felt across the front of Bev's abdomen, and things didn't look too promising. He was a pretty big baby---even allowing for the fact that he had a high head, he reached right up under Bev's ribs. A discussion of the likely outcome, transfer to base hospital for induction, plus the probable 'cascade of intervention', resulted in Bev deciding to have a try at persuading her baby to turn. Bev also decided to try the homoeopathic regime, as an added help.

She and the midwife worked out a plan of ways to make the baby uncomfortable in his present position, so that he would want to turn. Bev took a rocker home with her and sat on it straight away. It felt uncomfortable, as baby's weight was too far back in his present position. Bev found things easier when she put the rocker next to the table, as she could lean forward onto it. Still, the idea was to make him want to move, so Bev persevered. She began the homoeopathy and waited.

Late in the afternoon, her legs were getting puffy, so she went to bed for a rest. She took all the pillows, and arranged them so that she could lie on her front. This created a deep hammock and removed the support baby was getting from her abdominals. He didn't like that and began to turn. During the night there was furious activity in Bev's abdomen, and when she got up, she was a totally different shape!!

She came back to see the midwife at morning teatime saying,
"I hate you. I've had a terrible night". However, all the midwife said was "I'm sure you do, but just look at what's happened. Your baby has completely rotated!"

Bev went off to try and catch up on some sleep, and the midwife smiled as she waited for the next phase. Later that afternoon, Bev and her partner were back, labour going well, and just before supper a fine 4150g-baby girl was born. Bev was really pleased at how things had worked out for her, as she had expected at least forceps or quite possibly a caesarian section if her baby failed to move. It was a much more dramatic result than usual, as most first babies take a couple of days at least to turn.

The midwife's role

As you can see, once the parents had been provided with good information and had discussed ways to help themselves, there was again little to do, other than the required observations and their recording. Once the baby had turned, he was able to enter his mother's pelvis, flex his head well, and get himself born.

His mother's tissues were definitely more relaxed than usually happens when the baby is badly positioned until such a late stage of pregnancy. So this birth was the result of hard work on the part of the mother, coupled with a large dose of good fortune!

A Successful Home Birth After All

Joy's Story

Joy had planned to have her first baby at home so that she could control what was done to her. Everything went well until 38 weeks, when her baby had failed to assume the L O A position. She went to antenatal clinic to see an obstetrician, who after examining her and feeling the size of her baby said "You will never have this baby vaginally. I will book for a caesarian section next week before the baby is too big".

This really upset Joy, and she went home visibly troubled. Her partner and midwife were supportive and felt that the decision had been made too quickly. Joy was not a large woman, but neither was she very small. She also appeared to have a gynaecoid pelvis, so should be fine if her baby would move. The problem was that he had managed to get his head into the pelvis, and it was going to take a major effort by all involved if he was to be persuaded to turn. Joy went back to see the specialist, and told him that she was not going to have a caesarian until she had tried seriously to change things. She agreed to have non-stress monitoring each day---fortunately her home was close to the unit!

Now it was "all hands to the pumps". Joy spent most of each day on a rocker, with her knees well spread to make as much space as she could. For variety, she crawled round the floor with her nephew, and did sessions of "cat arches" to make the baby feel insecure. She pushed his pushchair down to the shops and back again a couple of times a day. At night, she slept with every pillow she could find under her head and legs, and between bosom and bulge.

Three days later nothing had happened. The baby kept making efforts to turn but didn't seem to be able to get round. Everyone was getting tired, but Joy was determined. The obstetrician was getting cross, and tried hard to insist on operating. However the baby seemed fine --there was no medical indication for hurry. Joy kept trying, and needed lots of help to resist the pressure from the unit.

Things stayed the same for another week, and even the midwife was feeling the disapproval from her peers.

Then just when Joy had been told that she was on her own, and that if she had to have an emergency caesarian the duty doctor would do it, things took a turn for the better. At last the baby managed to get right round !!!

Joy went into labour during the night, and after a solid 4 hour labour her 3955gram baby emerged--at home!

Maybe it would have been easier to "go with the flow" and have the caesarian section, but things were carefully monitored, and the baby was fine. He would certainly have found it easier to turn if he'd still been above the pelvic brim when Joy decided not to accept the obstetrician's advice.

The midwife's role

It was very stressful for her midwife, who was new to independent practice, and was harassed by the unit staff for failing to persuade Joy to follow the normal route. However, there were no real indications for intervention, so she felt her role was to monitor carefully, and be prepared to move to hospital at the first sign that things were not going well.

It was surprising that the baby's head was able to mould so well, as he was postmature.

Placental Site Nuisances

Karen's Story

Karen had felt for some weeks that her baby was not behaving in the way she expected. There were no definite humps and bumps in her abdomen when her baby moved. In fact she wasn't always sure that he was moving. She and her midwife checked her scan report---one of the times a scan proved useful. Yes, there it was, an anterior placenta, fairly low down as they often appear before the lower uterine segment develops. It was decided that although the baby would probably be facing forward, there was no point in trying to move him before 37/38 weeks, as until then there wouldn't be enough clear space for him to turn into. Like most babies, he was curled up facing his placenta, so the sponge like texture of the placenta muffled the movements Karen felt. It was easy to listen to the uterine souffle, and baby's heart was heard right round on Karen's right flank.

Karen prepared to wait a while, and eventually focused on the forward postures several times a day. It wasn't till around 39 weeks that her baby decided to move himself and stay put as an O A. Once he seemed settled, Karen wore a maternity girdle, to make it more difficult for him to change his mind, but he stayed O A, and was finally born on time + 3 days with minimal help from anyone but Mum.

The midwife's role

Karen's midwife <u>listened carefully</u> to her misgivings, <u>and responded</u> by checking the scan report. Once Karen had the situation explained, she understood that with her help, the baby would turn as the lower uterine segment grew.

A Cautionary Tale

<u>Debbie's Story</u>

Debbie was 38/40 weeks pregnant with her first baby, and having given up work, was enjoying some free time. She had a large baby on board, but she was a well built, well shaped lass, so expected things to go well. She also had a small car, quite old, with bucket seats. Her baby was not engaged, but he was vertex L O L and had his back properly placed.

One morning she and her mother decided to travel to a town about

100km away for a day out and to visit an aunt. As we've said, her baby was largish, and even with the seat pushed back, and a cushion to help her reach the pedals, Debbie didn't leave a lot of space for baby. All went well for the first 60 odd kilometres, and then baby got fed up with having his head squashed into the angle of Mum's pelvis and spine. He began to move strongly, and Debbie put up with it for a while, hoping he'd settle, but not understanding what he was upset about. Eventually, driving became too difficult, so she pulled over to the roadside and stopped. She stayed put as the activity got more vigorous in her abdomen, until finally after about half an hour it stopped. She set off again, and baby stayed quiet.

The next day, she realised that she was a totally different shape, and the baby's movements had changed. She came to the local unit, where a check revealed that her lovely O A was now definitely a breech!!! Despite everyone's best efforts, there was no way that baby would change back, so as was the custom at that time, Debbie went to the base hospital, and at due date was delivered by elective caesarian section.

The great pity was that if she had got out of her car and either walked about, or leant on the car with her tummy down the baby would have calmed down and stayed put. He couldn't stand the restriction on his head when Debbie was sitting with her knees raised and bottom low squashing him.

Most modern cars have seats that cause drivers to sit like this, so if a long journey must be taken, someone else should do the driving. It would be good if it would work the other way round, but it probably wouldn't, as the breech is so much smaller than the head.

Avoiding A Caesarian Section For Unstable Lie

Babies may choose to lie in positions from which they cannot enter the mother's pelvis. They may be facing backwards, but have their heads on one side, and their backs too straight. The commonest is the "Unstable Lie" where the head is merely tilted into mother's groin. Much more challenging is the Transverse Lie, where the baby lies across the abdomen with his lower shoulder over the inlet. Unless these babies can be persuaded to move, an elective caesarian is the norm.

These are almost always found in the abdomens of multips whose uterine and abdominal muscles have been well stretched. They are not common, but we need to think about them. Many professionals are frightened at the discovery. The truth is, that because a healthy cord floats, there is rarely a prolapse. Furthermore, how can he squash it if he's above the brim? If he descends, still facing backwards, his cord will tend to fit into one of the deep curves on either side of the sacral prominence.

It would have to get between his head or chest and the prominence to be squashed. Therefore as long as the membranes are intact, there is little likelihood of the cord being compressed between the baby's head and the pelvic floor. *Early ruptured membranes and a prolapsed cord are a definite emergency*. However, it is better to be safe than sorry, so we will look at ways to help before labour starts.

How To Help

What has happened, in most cases, is that instead of the baby's head being kept more or less in the middle, his bottom has moved too far to the side, and he's not curled up enough. This puts him in a diagonal or oblique angle to the pelvic inlet, instead of straight above it. If he's a shoulder presentation, he's lying on his side. Interestingly, he will almost always be facing mother's back---that relaxed hammock again !!

As the Braxton Hicks contractions increase in late pregnancy, the uterine muscle tone improves. This on its own may be enough. This mother will benefit immensely from wearing a well-fitting maternity girdle. When they were in common use, more babies stayed where they should. The new maternity pull-on girdle should be put on either before rising from bed or whilst leaning forward. It is elasticated at base and sides, thus providing a firm support for the uterus. The baby then finds it easier to assume the desired L O A position.

A Baby in the Oblique Position

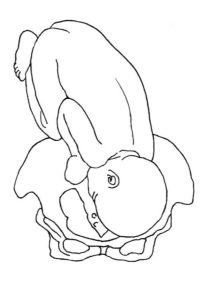

Dr. Buist described an old-fashioned (and much cheaper) idea that can often work.

Needed:

- One long binder or narrow towel
- Two standard towels
- Five safety pins

Procedure:

- With mother lying on her back, position binder under mother between ribs and thighs.
- Roll one towel into a sausage and place between right hip bone and uterus. (This tips baby's bottom straight.) Mother holds in place.
- Second towel is rolled and placed on left side. (This moves the head towards the centre.)Mother holds in place.
- Now wrap binder around and pin firmly at base and progressively more loosely above.

It is now worn for 24 hours, and will in most cases have done its job. Some women may need to continue to wear a girdle while up and about.

This will work when the mother is in niggly preparatory labour. In fact it is very useful at that time. An unstable lie due for caesarian can often is converted in a very short time, as the contractions are quite strong. The binder is applied, and the mother mobilised so that she is able to bend forward with each tightening.

This simple action saves an enormous amount of work, and causes no complications, as long as the membranes are intact. It should not be tried if they have ruptured.

<u>*Supporting, not compressing the Pregnant Abdomen*</u>

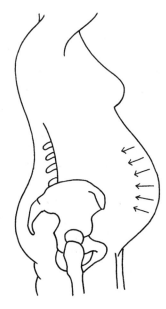 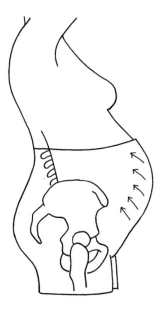

Don't tuck tail in to avoid backache.

Wear a Maternity Girdle.

A Couple Of Examples

Louise's Story (1)

Louise, gravida 4 para 3 came to a small unit one morning with erratic annoying contractions. Examination found an unstable lie, baby's head being in Louise's left groin area, and easily moved. The membranes were still intact. The idea of transfer to base hospital was resisted, as the other children were to be present to see the new brother or sister born. It was decided that an attempt would be made with towels and binder to coax the baby's head to engage. Louise was trussed up, a rolled towel on either side of her uterus and a binder pinned firmly holding them in place. Fortunately the baby was co-operative and straightened up as the binder was applied. Louise spent the next half- hour alternating between upright and forward leaning postures, as her contractions rapidly established. Baby stayed centred, and soon had her head engaged. A couple of hours later she made her appearance, much to the family's delight.

For most multips, it is only necessary to persuade the baby's head to angle directly onto the maternal cervix for results to be almost instantaneous. If attempts are made before the Braxton-Hicks contractions become strong, many babies will revert to the oblique when the binder is removed.

A Really Dramatic Affair

Les's Story (2)

Les. was 37 weeks pregnant with her third baby when she visited the unit with a baby who was quite definitely not lined up. A palpation found a transverse lie, but even worse, a shoulder already well into the brim. Les had had two very traumatic births in another part of the country. She had begun labour in small units, but been transferred to base hospitals, where major interventions had occurred. She was very anxious to have things go really well this time.

Just what was happening was carefully explained to Les and her husband. The baby was unable to lift his shoulder out of mother's pelvis to let his head in. The midwife described various postures, such as knee-chest, or lying on the back with a couple of pillows under the buttocks that might help. She also informed them of a homoeopathic regime that had been successful on other occasions. Les was asked to return in a few days. These things aren't always dramatic or instant.

When they returned the baby was still transverse--no change at all. The midwife could only say "It hasn't worked, so we'll have to book you for a caesarian at base." The response was dramatic---that was something Les would not have!! The midwife again explained just where the baby was lying, and asked Les to tell her how she thought the baby could get out of such a position. A short pause for thought, and Les asked for the information to be repeated. This was done, and a further supply of homoeopathics given. (These were not taken).

Les went home, determined to give the baby as much room as possible.

Next morning she rang to say, "It's turned, and I can feel its bottom under my ribs." Persuading her to share what she had done wasn't easy, but finally she described lying on her back on the floor with her knees hung over the back of the couch, and her bottom supported by pillows. No result from the first try but on the second, Les felt her baby drop back into her abdomen; a great heave and he was laying lengthways. When Les stood up she could feel baby's head drop through the brim of the pelvis at last.

Determined, Les also decided to wear a pair of maternity pantyhose during the day, but they were probably unnecessary, as by now Braxton Hicks contractions were toning up her uterus. She also kept a small pillow under her abdomen at night to help keep baby in the midline. Her reward was a due date arrival of a 3780g baby after a short labour at the small unit. Everyone was thrilled.

What was so interesting was that Les had not absorbed any of the first session. She expected the midwife to enable her to have the birth she wanted, without any input from her. The reality of a booking for a caesarian section, changed the whole picture, and Les realised that only she could affect the way her birth went.

She was also lucky that she began trying at a fairly early stage, as a spontaneous rupture of membranes when baby is transverse, and the mother is an hour or so away from effective help is a major emergency. It would have been much kinder to the small unit staff if the efforts had been made with Les much closer to the base hospital.

A Baby in the Transverse Position

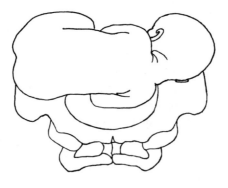

Section Five

Occipito Posterior Positions

- He is the baby who causes the long painful "entering pains" for the same reason.
- He provides very poor signals to his mother's body to prepare for his exit.

When labour eventually begins -

- His membranes will have ruptured early, and he will have lost any freedom of movement.
- He presses constantly against his mother's spine causing real discomfort.
- His bottom is brought forward as proper labour contractions begin. (These change the shape of the uterus and bring its top forward).
- He is able to start to enter the pelvis, but is still unable to flex properly.
- He moves down slowly---all the contraction pressure is exerted through his front onto the lower uterine segment instead of the cervix.
- His head stays in the oblique angle of his mother's pelvis, so the full length/depth of his head must descend.
- He is unable to use the sacral curve---if he does, he becomes a face presentation.
- He must reduce his head circumference to pass the "spines" and this takes time.
- He needs the cervix to dilate more than 10cm to exit the uterus-- again slow and painful.
- He is unable to rotate his shoulders at the pelvic brim as he can't get them far enough forward of the sacral prominence.

The "Rest And Be Thankful" Stage

This mother desperately needs the rest and be thankful stage to enable her baby to enter the cavity where there is room to rotate.
The mother needs a pause while she recharges her batteries.
Some mothers may need food, or a short sleep.

During Second Stage Labour –

His posterior shoulder is on the wrong side of the sacral prominence, and it is easy for his anterior shoulder to fix at the top of the symphasis.

- He will need to be pushed down by his mother. The back pain continues as he has the back of his neck against the sacrum and is still trying to rotate his shoulders. As it is difficult to push without a resistance to push against, every effort *must* be made to help the baby turn.

- The mother needs to keep her weight forward to help him turn-- Lying down is not wise, but in this case a few contractions while on the right side may help. This uses his body weight to help him straighten. How his head will be born--normally, face to pubes, or obliquely will be determined by the position of his shoulders. His neck is flexible, but he can't twist his head right round.

  He may:
- Turn his head across the pelvis and become arrested (transverse arrest at the spines).
- Pass the spines and rotate on the pelvic floor, also managing to sort his shoulders out at the brim, becoming a normal O.A.

99

- Continue to descend facing forward and will be born as a "face to pubes" or direct O.P.
- Fail to rotate his shoulders at the brim and is unable to descend without medical help. It is very difficult for him to bring his posterior shoulder across the sacral promontory.

Post Natally -

- The baby will be unhappy and very tired because of the long birth process.

- He will need treating as if he has concussion (which in effect he has).

- Feeding may be difficult if his hypoglossal nerve has been pinched---he will be unable to use his tongue properly.

For the mother -

- Perineal discomfort may be severe.

- Confident handling of her baby may take longer to establish.

- She may need extra support   "I couldn't mother my baby because I needed someone to mother me".

The OP Baby has his head erect as in the "Military" Position

Foetal Heart at 'x'

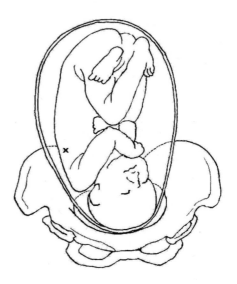

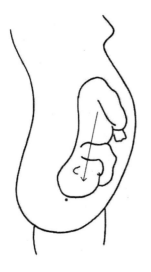

Contractional Pressure is 2-3cm in front of the cervix therefore the cervix does not dilate as effectively

<u>*Who is Affected by an O.P ?*</u>

This is the situation that left uncorrected causes almost all our problems. *Everyone is affected.*

- *The mother,* as she experiences the sheer awfulness of an O.P. baby trying to prepare for and complete the process of labour and birth. It is a real endurance test, even with all the modern support systems of pain relief. No woman should be asked to suffer in this way, when so many can be helped, by good midwifery interventions.

  Must she suffer the discomfort, or pain above and behind her pubes as baby tries at every chance to rotate? The sets of contractions, that can be so regular and pronounced that she feels "it must be real labour". The disturbed sleep, that brings her to labour already worn out. Experiencing the constant backache of labour that becomes worse with each contraction.

These can all be resolved, if the baby and mother work together to help him reposition himself.

- *The baby,* as its head is subjected to unnatural forces throughout the whole process. If we were unable to rescue them, many of today's infants would suffer serious brain damage. Tentorial tears may be uncommon, but how many of the children we know with dyslexia, attention deficit disorder, varying degrees of lack in physical coordination, from clumsiness to inability to take part in everyday play, glue ear, poor eyesight,. etc…. had a "Bad Birth?" How many of the colicky babies, the poor feeders, and so on till the list is frightening?

If we looked at them, we would probably find almost all them had some deviation from the normal process.

- ***The midwife and support people,*** as they try to relieve the mother's pubic pain when the baby tries harder to enter the pelvis. The result is that even before real labour starts everyone is tired and vulnerable. It is no wonder we look for ways to provide rapid relief, or that mothers are so welcoming of epidurals!

- ***The hospital,*** as so much of its Maternal and Childcare budget is used to provide the extra attention these mothers and their babies need. Delivery suites--that phrase again! Special care nurseries, for the hypoglycaemic, stressed out newborns; all gobble up large sums that could be better spent on support services for new mothers, if the rate of normal births was increased.

Midwives have a responsibility to rediscover the ways to keep birth normal for everyone's sake. We get only one chance at being born. There are no rehearsals, no second chances. It must be right first time.

Midwives have been so busy becoming a profession that we have given too little attention to our other important role.

We are the ones who "Stand With Women", giving them the knowledge and support they need. There is no place in Midwifery for people who make women dependent on them. That is what is wrong with today's Obstetrics. It is designed to put the professional in the leading role. It can't be otherwise while so many women are unable to give birth by their own efforts, but many of the problems are created by the very system set up to prevent them.

The public are obviously concerned. Most Western countries have their own version of the Cumberledge Report. It sounds great, but what will have changed in 5 years?

The "warm fuzzies", or extra personal attention, will for a while blind women to the fact that all that has changed is that they are now dependent on the Midwife, rather than the doctor. Will the types and outcomes of labour and birth have altered? I doubt it.

Our whole training needs reviewing, as do almost all our textbooks.

Why do O.P.s find being born so difficult?

To answer that question, we need to go back to our first anatomy lesson.

Let's consider the pelvis once again.- Most of our new textbooks treat the female pelvis as a static passage. Not true. They also depict it as almost level at the brim especially when the baby is included. Also not true.

When we are standing, our sacrum is much higher than our symphasis--in fact, the angle is 120" or more. The curve of the female sacrum is very pronounced, bringing the coccyx level with the middle of the symphasis, rather than the base, as in the male pelvis. The effect of pregnancy lordosis in increasing the distance between the maternal sacrum and symphasis is rarely, if ever, mentioned. We seem to have difficulty accepting that for a normal birth, the baby's back needs to be swung forward, supported by his mother's abdominal muscles, if he is to get his posterior parietal under her sacrum. The text is often fine, but who checked the drawings? Admittedly, it is hard to draw from a frontal angle.

Pelvimetry is used to answer the wrong questions. There are very, very, few women today with a deficient pelvis. Even large babies i.e. around 4000-4500 gm will fit IF their mothers keep leaning forwards.

The available space of the pelvis in the resting state bears little resemblance to that available as a birthing mother swings her weight from one foot to the other, bends her knees, or performs the active response to her baby's demands that a well informed mobile mother does. The bones themselves cannot open, during first stage but the space is increased in the diameter matching the raised leg.

Birth is a dynamic happening, not a passive endurance test as we are being taught.

Where are we taught about the "rhombus of Michaelis " and its role in physiological second stage labour? Some old textbooks mention the extra available space as something that happens as a matter of course. How could it have been forgotten?

Did the availability of supposedly safe analgesia, followed by even stronger anaesthesia, cause us to lose our instinctive knowledge? Or did we women grab their availability with both hands as we dropped the responsibility for our safety and that of our babies? Was it because with O.A. babies, the process is empowering, or was it because by getting women to "leave it to us dear" so many people gained power, prestige, and job satisfaction?

Whatever the reasons, and I guess they are as varied as the practitioners, the end result, especially for the babies has been disastrous. Once the interior of their heads has been distorted by unnatural angles of pressure during the birth process, there is no mechanism to restore it. In a normal birth, the suckling at the breast, as well as the baby's crying realign any deviations. For the O.P.

baby, none of this makes any difference. Their mothers are often totally demoralised as the expected simple birth is transformed into yet another medical rescue, and in many cases are only too happy to transfer the care of their young to nurseries or daycare. Many lay people are trying hard to help the recovery by women of their natural function, but without our help they have a long, hard road to travel.

To continue.....

The O.P. baby has his head erect, as in the "Military " position. That describes it very well. In this position, he has his back in the curve of his mother's hip, almost always the right. We discussed why earlier, but here it is again. The full term uterus has a distinct lean to the right. It is also turned slightly to the left at the base. Correctly, a right obliquity, and dextro-rotation. The mother's stomach, colon and rectum on the left side also tend to push baby to her other side if he is facing forward.

The Primigravid uterus is pear shaped, so there is not much room in the lower segment for the baby's head to lie in an R.O.A. angle. As we know, the Multip has an apple shaped uterus, so her baby may enter the pelvis as R O L and then choose R.O.A. The birth then follows the normal pattern.

If he remains an O P, the baby is presenting with the full vertex. This measures between 35.5 and 37cm in circumference. It has an Occipito-frontal length of 11.5cm in most cases. This will fit, if the neck is able to bend, allowing the head to fit under the maternal sacrum. That is a very rare pre-labour happening today for a normal sized baby. The curve of his mother's lumbar spine, plus the forward protrusion of her sacrum, combine to keep him high, straight, and above the brim. If most of his mother's time is spent sitting the distance between her spine and symphasis is even less than the

9.5cm of his bi-parietal. There is just no way he can enter the maternal pelvis. Added to this is the discomfort felt by the mother, every time her baby tries to move.

Entering Pains

Unlike normal Braxton-Hicks contractions, the ones triggered by the baby trying to turn may continue for up to 15-20 minutes! This is an unmanageable length of time by any standards, though so often the poor mother is told "it's just baby trying to engage." She already knows that. It is her bladder and symphasis that are being assaulted. No, that is not too strong a term. Women remember the pain many years later. Most mothers try to relieve the pain by lifting the abdomen and uterus upwards, thus ensuring that the baby is unsuccessful and will have to try again.

The whole exhausting process may continue off and on for several weeks, with the baby trying harder, and the mother being worn out. A great way to start on an O.P. labour. that could last for days. No wonder mothers are receptive to the idea of induction, epidural, and all over within 12 hours.

During Birth

During the birth, the O P baby's head remains upright, and the contraction force travelling down his front is unable to push him into the sacral curve. (The few who do use all the space present as faces.) The maximum pressure is at a point around 2-3cm in front of the maternal cervix, so dilation is even slower than expected. The effacement stage is seriously prolonged, as there is little or no effective pressure on the cervix. The baby must contend with the lack of liquor, whether this was spontaneous or induced. The lack of it certainly makes things harder. In addition, if he's to pass the ischial spines he must reduce his head circumference from 35.5 - 37cm by changing the shape of the parietals, which takes time. Either that or he'd have grooves down both sides of his head.

If he is still in the transverse when he reaches the "spines", as so many of them are, he cannot escape but becomes a transverse arrest, needing a Caesarian section, or Keiland's forceps rotation to survive.

He is again in trouble at the outlet if he fails to rotate on the pelvic floor. There is plenty of room for a nicely flexed O.A., but the O.P. has large diameters trying to distend the perineum, and unless his mother is able to bend her knees and arch her back--thus providing the extra space, he is likely to be caught.

Obviously, he must move his face along the inside of the pubes before any second stage progress is possible, and this needs a lot of pushing by his mother. How can he turn his shoulders across the back of the pelvis to pass the sacral prominence?

The practice of putting mothers to bed, and then asking them to raise their legs during second stage labour is ridiculous.

This is so true. It dramatically increases the Curve of Carus, while pulling the large glutoid muscles tight, meaning that the Rhomboid of Michaelis, (that diamond shaped area including the sacral prominence) is unable to move backwards as it should.

Even worse is the practice of using stirrups. The need for forceps deliveries (that word again) could be reduced almost to nil if instead of trying to turn the baby, the mother was encouraged to change her position.

Some old textbooks, discussing failure to progress in second stage, advocate placing the mother across the bed, legs hanging, and placing two firm pillows under the buttocks. Just like an upright mother allowing her abdomen to sag downwards. Amazing!!!

Mobile or Bedridden O.P labour?

What happens during the labour and birth is quite different when the mother is upright and mobile from the sequence if she is bedridden, so we must look at them independently.

First, we need to consider the things they have in common.

Firstly, postmaturity is a feature. The baby's placenta is ageing, and his head is ossifying. Both are likely to make a bad situation worse. The ability of the head to mould is greatly reduced.

Secondly, the membranes usually rupture early. There is usually a longish time--up to several days--as the uterine muscles adapt to the smaller internal volume. Contractions may commence spontaneously, or syntocinon may be used. The baby loses the support and protection of the liquor as he tries to rotate.

Thirdly, if labour starts it is often erratic, with bouts of contractions, close together, for several hours and then fading out. This may go on before as well as after the membranes rupture.
Sometimes there is just a hindwater leak, but in all cases the mother feels unpleasantly damp at all times. She also feels worse as liquor oozes past the head with movement or contractions.

The major similarity is the type and frequency of the contractions. Too many,- too close,- too painful. The constant backache is also morale shattering.

The "Normal" Sequence

First we will look at the way the foetal head and maternal pelvis interact in a mobile unrestricted birth.

The first sign that labour is imminent is often a spontaneous membrane rupture (S R M).

Contractions may not start for some time, as the uterine muscles adapt to the loss of tension when the liquor drains out. This stage is also often ignored when a mother's labour is induced.

In a normal situation, once a check has been made that the baby's cord has not prolapsed, the mother should remain mobile. She needs to be able to constantly adjust the internal diameters of her pelvis as her baby moves. ***Her posture affects the way the whole birth will go.***

The baby's erect head may enter the pelvis once labour contractions start. These tilt the top of the uterus forward   bringing the baby's bottom forward with it, so that after a while, the baby's head may have bent enough to enter the brim. As it moves down through the pelvis, still upright, it is able to use only a small part of the space.

The pressure from contractions is through the baby's front, so loses much of its power. What remains reaches the lower uterine segment, rather than the cervix.

In most cases, the contractions are closely spaced from the start. Three minutes apart and 40-50 seconds long. The head is pressed against the maternal sacral prominence, so the pain never fades but is ever present, becoming worse during each contraction.

Eventually, the head is moulded enough to pass out of the fully dilated cervix into the vagina. Now it passes the ischial spines, and is able to rotate against the pelvic floor into the O.A. position. From here a normal birth takes place.

All this takes longer than where the baby begins as O.A. Its success within a reasonable time frame depends on the mother responding to the internal pressures and pains she feels.

Special attention needs to be paid to the mother's fluid and electrolyte levels if she is to have the stamina to continue. Low blood sugars and calcium levels mean a much lower pain tolerance.

What else may happen?

The badly directed contraction force may have several unwanted effects.

It may stretch the lower segment of the uterus until the less experienced of us think that full dilation has occurred. This is a not uncommon situation! A V.E. by a more experienced midwife discovers a cervix very posterior, and not even effaced. At other times there may be sufficient strength to dilate the cervix to around 5cm before ceasing, when the diagnosis is "failure to progress".

If the baby's head remains in the transverse, there is little or no moulding despite almost continuous contractions. There is constant pressure on the maternal sacrum, with backache that is always present, and gets worse with each contraction.

If the baby moves to the oblique, he will be able to move further down the pelvic cavity, and if his head moulds enough he will be able to pass the "spines." From there, if he's lucky, he may rotate on the pelvic floor to O.A. and be born by his own and his mother's efforts.

Again he may get out "face to pubes". This is not a good fit, but by much pushing and shoving by mother, he may be born. The pressure is on the pelvic floor instead of in front of it. This means that in most cases an episiotomy or tear will enlarge the outlet.

Many babies fail to emerge in a reasonable time, as the angle of force is incorrect and there is nothing in the cavity for it to work against. The baby just stays put. His shoulders are at the wrong angle to the pelvic brim, so fail to enter. The mother must make enormous efforts at pushing, but these may well be useless.

It is the O.P. baby who needs "rescuing" by forceps or caesarian. His size is irrelevant. A 2900gm baby in the transverse will fail to progress, where a 4000gm O.A. would have plenty of room in the same pelvis.

There is only one angle at which all the space can be utilised, and that is the O.A.

All these troubles are magnified if the mother is confined to bed. The mother's back is rounded, so the pressure angle is even more inefficient. The mother is sitting on her sacral curve instead of her ischial tuberosities, thus bringing her spine and symphasis too close. The main pelvic floor muscles are behind the ischial spines, so there is maximum pelvic floor resistance. In front, the only obstacle is the bladder, and that should be empty. The spacing of contractions and the uphill angle mean that the baby has no chance to rotate in the cavity.

How can we help?

These are the babies and mothers that really need our expert help. *We can prevent almost all O.P. labours, if we concentrate our efforts on the Antenatal period.*

Most women attend their clinic, G.P. or Midwife regularly over the last few weeks of pregnancy. Never mind that they come hoping to be told when it will be over! We do see them.

What do we find? - -The usual signs of an O.P.-- High, flat abdomen, small parts i.e. the arms and legs towards the mother's front, the baby's back far out on the right. The heartbeat is most easily heard in the right flank, and if the valves are to be located they will be hard to find.

This position is of no real significance before 36weeks for a primigravida, or up to 39 for a multigravida.

After this it is important that the mother, and her support team, understand why the baby must be persuaded to turn.

This is time consuming, so we need to be involved with the antenatal education in our area. The mothers don't come? If what they want is provided there is no problem. It is when we decide what is good for them that they stay away in droves.

Everyone is interested in how birth happens. Men find the technical details of "how the bits fit" fascinating. They are also not pregnant, so can take in the details. Most first time Mums just want it over, with as little discomfort as possible. They are looking for ideas on how to shorten the process.

If it is explained that a baby in the right position, has his head down and his back on Mum's left, between her hip and umbilicus, the majority of parents work things out for themselves. Partners encourage proper postures, for resting and sleeping.

Everyone watches to see how baby's position changes. If it is painful, as it can be, there is support. For many women, there is far more pain in the week before the birth than during it. The worst part is that there is no pattern to when they occur or how long the baby's efforts last.

It is even worse if the baby is still high and trying to turn after the membranes rupture. Added to this is the idea of counting and timing contractions.

Who ever first taught them that when contractions are 5 minutes apart, it is time for hospital?

Maybe it's okay for O.A.s as they have close contractions for a relatively short time. Most mothers are quite sure by then that they are in labour. Pity the poor lass with an O.P. She will have close contractions right through the preparatory stage. If she starts counting, by the time labour really starts she is exhausted from discomfort and lack of sleep.

Section Six

Some Interesting
O.P Stories

Section Six: Some Interesting OP Stories

"Once again the midwife is the protector of the birthing family."

There are so many possible scenarios for an O.P. labour and birth, that it will be easiest to treat them as "birth stories" and follow them through the process.

All these mothers came to labour with their babies still un-rotated. That is, still lying on the mother's right side, with back between her spine and hip. They were mostly postmature, and likely to experience the full O P birth.

Spontaneous Rotation on the Pelvic Floor

Shelley's Story

Shelley arrived at delivery suite (that phrase again) with spontaneous rupture of membranes at 41 weeks. Everything was fine, except that her baby was R.O.P. engaged, with a badly fitting presenting part.

There was no cord felt, so she remained upright and mobile. Her baby was quite active, but there were no contractions. Her midwife felt that walking up and down the corridors would have little effect, but suggested trying going quietly up and down a few flights of stairs.

Shelley soon tired of this and decided that her partner should go home for some much-needed sleep and she would go to bed. As her baby was on her right side, she lay on her left, to see if he would turn. A pillow between bed and body helped with the drag on her abdominal muscles. She did get 2 hours sleep, which was to be invaluable later on.

Fortunately contractions began before syntocinon was started. They were strong, and close from the start, causing Shelley to wonder if she would be able to handle them.

Progress was slow, effacement being finally complete 10 hours after S.R.M. Syntocinon was started, and shortly afterwards, an epidural anaesthetic begun. Shelley was now confined to bed, but remained on her left side. She was unable to pass urine, so had to be catheterised-- something she found humiliating.

The syntocinon rate had to be increased to maximum before dilatation became steady.

Finally full dilatation was reached, and the epidural was allowed to decrease to give Shelley a chance to push her baby out. The baby's head met the pelvic floor, and during a contraction, it began to turn. Shelley stayed on her side, so that her pelvic outlet was level and able to open as the baby came down. She rotated her right hip upwards and outwards as the midwife told her that she could see baby finishing the turn. Baby Joe appeared, head very well moulded, but in the O.A. position. There was a small tear as Joe brought both shoulders out at the same time.

The midwife's role

Shelley needed a great deal from her midwife.

She had been to classes, where everything focussed on birth as a normal female act, and everyone made wonderful birth plans. She found the information that her baby was posterior hard to accept. If she had known earlier why she was getting so much supra-pubic pain she would have been happier. Now that she was faced with a long and probably painful labour, she had no plan to cope.

Shelley felt let down by the system and it took quite some time for her to accept that there was no failure in taking advantage of pain relief, especially once syntocinon was in use.

Apart from helping Shelley to understand that it was not her fault that her baby had chosen the O.P. position, the midwife had to help her partner find ways to provide the extra support needed as she dealt with her lost dream.

It was a bonus that the baby turned, and was born by his and Shelley's efforts, as many women are not so fortunate, and carry a burden of feeling a failure with them into motherhood.

These are the mothers that need so much help but are so emotionally draining of their midwife. They also need a really good support system to be able to keep giving to those who need them, not least their new born babies.

An Extra Special Midcavity Spontaneous Rotation
(You can't be right all the time!)

Cherry's Story

Cherry had been labouring well for several hours with her first baby. The small unit was quiet, as the midwives changing shifts discussed each mother's progress. The night midwife felt that Cherry should have a V.E., but the room seemed so full of positive signs that the oncoming midwife was reluctant.

However Cherry wanted to know how long it would be, and the records needed updating. So a V.E. was carried out. It revealed a midline cervix, at 5cm dilation, and an anterior fontanelle right there.

Cherry was given two scenarios. If she was prepared to be mobile and the baby moved position, then perhaps the baby would be born around lunchtime. Otherwise, early evening seemed more realistic.

Duties at the postnatal end of the hospital called, and Cherry was left kneeling with her arms over her supporting aunts and wiggling her bottom.

Less than an hour later, an aunt appeared to tell the midwife that Cherry wanted to push! Of course the midwife made all the right comments about OP babies and premature pushing, but she felt she was missing something.

From the doorway of her room, Cherry could be seen moving both buttocks independently while holding the bed rail. It was clear that in this instance the baby was indeed coming.- A small 3000g baby slid onto the bed with no pushing at all.

The midwife was amazed, as she had never seen a primip go from 5cm dilated to delivered in such a short time (less than an hour!) It was definitely an advertisement for self directed movement during labour. It also gave Cherry a positive experience – one of very few in her short life.

The midwife's role

Apart from the checking of all recordings as well as the V.E. at the shift change, the midwife's role was minimal.

Cherry was well cared for by her family, and needed nothing from the midwife, who felt that she would be intruding if she stayed. She was very surprised at the speed of progress. Once Cherry knew how to help herself and her baby she applied the knowledge most effectively.

This birth was a real eye-opener for the midwife, who believed many things in an abstract way, but until now had failed to internalise them.

Complete failure of Midwifery Advice

The next Primigravida who arrived in so-called labour with an O.P. was completely different. She had no intention of helping herself, but expected her baby to be removed from her body with no help from his mother.

Belinda's Story

Belinda was having really nasty entering pains as her baby tried to get himself turned into her pelvis. She arrived with several family members, who were keen to help her have a normal birth.
However, Belinda had decided that she would be transferred to the base hospital, have an epidural and probably a caesarian section.

The midwife on duty tried hard to persuade her that it was much easier to do things herself, and that she would recover more quickly after a spontaneous birth and no stitches. Her family were supportive, and even tried to take Belinda home, to see if proper labour would start.

No way! Belinda sat firm on her low chair, knees above her seat and with her bottom lip stuck out. Her statement was, " I won't; you can't make me! " Of course she was right. So her doctor was contacted and off she went to the base hospital. She had her wish. ARM, syntocinon, epidural and caesarian section!

This was a dramatic example of a mother who had no desire to be involved with her birth process. What was behind it no-one ever knew, but there was absolutely no way she could be encouraged to help herself.

Face To Pubes

Anne's Story

Anne was 41+ weeks pregnant with her first baby. She had been having bouts of contractions, of erratic length and frequency for a week. These had been worse at night, as her baby tried to turn, and she had been out of bed several times a night. She had even been ready to go to hospital as they became regular and more painful. Each time they finally ceased, but she was worn out from lack of sleep. Eventually her membranes ruptured, but nothing more happened for 12 hours.

At last they began, but instead of short and widely spaced, they were 5 minutes apart, long, and very painful.

Her midwife checked that there is no cord presenting, so she remained mobile and at home. She ate a small meal- this was going to be a long process.

In the previous week, on midwife advice, she had bought some lemon and blackcurrant sweets to keep her (and as importantly) her baby's sugar levels up. Low blood sugar plus low calcium levels equals low pain tolerance. She had also made some concentrated fruit juice ice-cubes to refresh and sustain her.

With each contraction, Anne moved her hips from one side to the other. She wasn't keen on the idea of stair climbing but otherwise responsive to internal pressure.

Four hours later, the situation is,

- Presentation: Vertex
- Position: R.O.P
- Engagement: Complete
- Contractions: 1 x 3 lasting 40-50 seconds
- Dilation: 2cm
- Maternal condition: Distressed
- Foetal Heart: 140 strong regular
- **Decision:**   **Proceed to hospital for pain relief.**

Anne was prescribed a "walking" epidural, and was able to continue out of bed to full dilation. She maintained forward leaning postures, which allowed descent to proceed at a steady rate.

Her partner ensured that she emptied her bladder at regular intervals, thus keeping as much space as possible, and preventing damage to her bladder and urethra

She popped a sweet between her gum and cheek at 1/2 hourly intervals, to help keep herself independent. As the end of first stage approached, she used a straw to drink the small amount of ice cube that had melted during the contraction.

The urge to push before full dilation was lessened while Anne stayed mobile, and her midwife agreed that she should give birth kneeling over a beanbag on the end of the bed.

The movement of the sacral prominence was slight, as in all O.P. positions, so Anne had to actively push her baby down. She did well, and after 30 minutes, the baby's head became visible.

She was encouraged to arch her back, and take her weight on her folded lower legs. Her partner was standing at the end of the bed, so she held him around his neck for a more upright position

The baby pivoted against her pubes, and the top of its head, then its occiput appeared, followed by the back of its neck. As it extended the face was born, followed quickly by rotation and the birth of the posterior shoulder. The rest of the body was born, with no perineal damage.

This was a successful birth outcome for all involved.

The midwife's role

Once again the midwife was the protector of the birthing family. Too much contact, -back rubbing, applying cold cloths to Anne's forehead,- prevent the mother from entering the detached state of increased endorphin production that is needed if she is to succeed without chemical pain relief.

It is very hard for onlookers to see the apparent pain during contractions. They need the midwife's help to accept that each pain is short-lived, and that if Anne is able to respond to it she will manage well.

Time passes very quickly for labouring women, as their senses are totally focused on internal events. Eye contact is especially bad, as the mother finds herself "pulled" to the surface.

Anne wanted an epidural despite understanding about endorphins, but the amount was able to be kept to a minimum.

There was a need for closer monitoring but a portable sonicaid enabled this to be done without intruding into the mother's detached state.

Once again it is a case of "less is more" as the labour progresses faster and more smoothly when there are few other people disturbing the privacy.

Maybe this is where the idea that all midwives do is drink tea comes from.

There is an old and very wise saying—"When tempted to intervene, try sitting on your hands for 10 minutes!"—doesn't stop us observing, but gives the birth process a chance to change for the better.

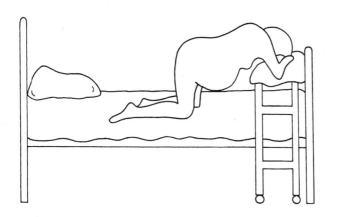

Labouring at the Foot End of the Bed will keep the Head End Clean

A Note for Midwives

Remember, Anne's midwife is seeing the birth from a totally different angle, to the view she would have if Anne were on her back.

The midwife lifts the baby and passes him between Anne's legs as she sits back on her heels.

Mother and baby are helped to sit back in the normal position at the head of the bed, where the cord is cut, and the placenta delivered.

Why choose the end of the bed?

When mothers give birth leaning over the top of the bed there is a major problem helping them turn to the usual position, against the pillows while the placenta is still undelivered, and the mother wants to hold her baby. For many of us, once is quite enough. Getting the incontinence sheet out and replaced, trying to avoid the "drips" from the placenta, etc. etc.-it all adds up to a messy situation, that few of us care to repeat.

From the end of the bed however, it's tuck the toes under, and straight back onto a clean bed. Much quicker and much easier.

Midcavity Rotation with Midwife Assistance

Kelly's Story

Kelly was hoping to have her second baby at home, but progress was slow. She'd had ruptured membranes for 12 hours, and was still only 5cm dilated. Contractions were 1 / 3 lasting 40 seconds. Backache was constant and not relieved by hot packs. Foetal heart-rate 132-140 variable. Vital signs normal.

Everything else was fine. Mother's condition was good and she was coping well. Fluid intake and output were stable. She ate tart glucose sweets regularly, to keep her own and baby's blood sugars up. Concentrated fruit juice ice-cubes were sucked between contractions for the same reason.

Kelly began to wonder if this home-birth idea was such a good one after all! She booked into the local unit "just in case". The prospect of relief from the constant backache and intense cervical pain with each contraction started to become more and more appealing.

Kelly, her partner and her midwife discussed the state of affairs. It seemed that there was still quite some way to go, as the baby was still behind the transverse. They had hoped that with Kelly mobile that it would have rotated.

Kelly's midwife had previously been successful in helping babies to rotate while doing a V.E. They agreed that the situation should be clarified so Kelly's midwife did a V.E. to help her decide what she wished to do. Her cervix was effaced, but still only 5cm dilated.

Kelly was lying on her back, which is not the most favourable position, but she agreed that for just three contractions her midwife would keep two opened fingers still and in place, although she was unable initially to reach the baby's head. As he was forced down by the contractions, the midwife's fingers provided a false pelvic floor. (If they are kept perfectly still, most babies will first do nothing but on the next contraction, will start to rotate.)

Kelly was made aware that there would be quite severe pain with each contraction, which is why she agreed to three only. In the middle of the third pain, the midwife felt the baby's head turn against her fingers, and Kelly said, " Thank goodness!"

The midwife removed her fingers and Kelly turned onto her knees to catch her breath.

From here, the normal O.A. process carried on and baby Jack was born in less than an hour.

Midwife's Role

Obviously the role of the midwife and her confidence and expertise were crucial in this situation.

The excellent relationship and evident trust between midwife and expectant parents was a major factor in determining this birth outcome.

Good communication and understanding of the birth process was also very important. Birthing mothers can withstand almost any pain as long as they know it is purposeful, productive and won't be endured for too long!

A Note For Midwives

This rotation is most effectively done with the mother either on all fours, leaning over pillows or a beanbag on the bed, or even standing.

A really determined baby has been known to need three fingers, and this is only tolerable in forward leaning positions.

It is quite hard for the midwife, as her hand is facing downward, and at the first few attempts, feels unnatural.

If it is done after full discussion with the mother, and the fingers are kept as still as possible, it is almost always successful.

It is especially useful where the mother is labouring at home, a birth centre or small unit, as once the baby has rotated, the birth process progresses well.

There is no point in trying, before 5cm, as the midwife's fingers are unable to open enough to form a false pelvic floor. At any later stage, even at full dilation with a transverse arrest it can work in spectacular fashion. On these occasions, it may be found that, with the mother in a forward leaning position, the midwife's fingers (pointing towards the sacrum) can apply gentle upward pressure between contractions, either side of the sagital suture to start the baby moving.

Transverse Arrest

Sally's Story

Sally was having her third baby in a small unit. All her babies had been large--around the 4000G size.

Progress was good, until second stage. Sally was in bed, on her back, with only 2 pillows. She had been pushing without effect for an hour, so her G P began the arrangements for transfer to the base hospital. Sally wasn't keen, as she had had no problems with the first two births.

Shift change, and the new midwife appeared. She didn't want to take an ambulance ride before breakfast. It would mean being away from the unit for three hours, and an on-call wasn't available.

The midwife and Sally held a discussion. It was suggested that Sally might like to get out of bed--an idea that horrified her husband. However, Sally needed no second telling and was out and leaning against the side of the bed in a flash.

It was fascinating to watch her contacting her baby. The expression on her face as she moved her body, increasingly with each contraction was amazing. Three went by, with Sally saying, "No, that's not it." In the middle of the fourth, a cry –
" Got it! " as the baby found room to move its head past the spines.

Sally fell onto the bed, and the baby came out, just as the ambulance trolley reached the door. Everyone was happy, including the husband!

While Sally was in bed with her knees up, every time she pushed, she jammed the baby's head tighter onto the spines.

Getting up, leaning forward and moving her pelvis gave the baby room to turn its head into the direct A P and pass the spines.

Midwife's Role

O.K. So timing and the overall needs of the unit definitely played a part in allowing Sally to give birth under her own efforts here. It's quite usual that we midwives respond well under such pressures, as in the previous example.

Perhaps it is precisely such time constraints and "resource" shortages that should be propelling us more and more towards encouraging the normal to remain normal, instead of opting for the medicalised alternatives quite so quickly!

Section Seven

Positions, Protocols
and Pain Relief

Section Seven: Positions, Protocols And Pain Relief

" The powerful, preconceived images, reinforced by the media, of labouring women lying down in bed to give birth must be understood and dispelled. "

Television dramas and literature mostly portray the idea of labouring women either lying on their backs or sitting on the floor against a sofa with knees raised and feet flat on the floor to give birth. They also portray the birth occurring after a few pushes and screams. Of course we know for the most part this is utter nonsense, but it looks good for dramatic purposes.

However we must be aware that this is precisely the visual image that most first time, novice mums have imbibed. (Many without even realising it.)

These powerful preconceived images, reinforced by the media, of labouring women lying down in bed to give birth must be understood if they're to be overcome and dispelled.

Futhermore, we have become so accustomed to labouring women going to bed, that we have come to believe that they are passive participants in the birth process. Somehow, we have also come to believe that the baby is only a passenger.

The choice of words by the first writers of textbooks has led us into a blind alley.

We have all stood beside a bed and explained to a mother that the pubic pain she is feeling is "only the baby turning." If that is so, just when does he stop participating? Many babies can be seen moving during labour. Some are extremely active right through, as if they can't wait to get out.

Would the process be clearer if we described birth as " **Letting the Baby out** "? In actual fact that is precisely what is happening. The mother's body is opening up to do just that.

Today's mothers are bombarded with advice on how to give birth normally, but how many of them achieve success?

And when they don't, no one tells them why they didn't. They are sometimes left with feelings of failure that may last a lifetime.

It is extremely rare for the mother to cause the failure if she has the information she needs. Once we have things clear in our own minds we can make a major contribution to increasing the rate of normal births either in our private practice, or for most of us in (that word again) "delivery" suite.

How and Why Being Bedridden Reduces the chance of a Normal Birth

Occipito Anterior

Being restricted to bed makes things hard even for the baby who is in a good position to start with. He needs to use the inward and backward slope of the symphasis to enable him to tuck his chin in.
When his mother is in bed, even propped up, she must keep her knees bent to stop herself slipping down the bed. She is now sitting on her sacral curve, rather than her ischial tuberosities. Instead of her sacral prominence being 6.5cm higher than the top of her symphasis, it is between 1 and 2cm.

This almost flat plane means that the baby's head remains at an upright angle. There is not enough space for the baby to slip its head under the sacrum and make use of all the room in the maternal pelvis.

The inner aspect of the ischia flare outwards and forward, providing no resistance for the baby's head to flex against.

Add to this, the exaggerated curve of the sacrum (the Curve of Carus) slowing down descent, and restricting the outlet and we can see where the need for all this orchestrated pushing comes from.

The action of the uterus is also badly compromised when the mother is reclining. If she is able to lean forward during contractions, things are much more efficient. The sides of the uterus tighten, the top flattens off, and the whole uterus tilts forward. Every scrap of energy is directed down baby's back and onto the cervix.

When she is reclining, a large part of the energy must be used to lift the uterus up and forward ("the uterus rears up" say the books.) What a waste of effort!

As the baby's head is not flexing properly, there is also muddled pressure on the cervix. This is why an anterior lip may happen on an apparently well fitting O.A. The head remains slightly straight, and there is a diameter of 11cm instead of 9.5cm trying to pass into the vagina. The cervix "catches" on the parietals.

Sometimes it can be slipped back--rather a painful happening for the mother, or she can be asked to turn onto her knees, which lifts the baby far enough off the cervix for its head to move. If the mother is a multip, there is usually a spectacular conclusion, as the baby makes his entrance into the world.

Second Stage

Having to push a baby into the world is another thing that has happened since mothers were put to bed to labour and be delivered. Babies can emerge unaided if the mother is on her side----it used to happen when chloroform put them to sleep. The second stages were not prolonged if the baby was the right way round.

The very worst thing that can happen is for the mother to be asked to bring her legs up around her abdomen to push. Placing them on the midwife's hips is also a not a good idea. How are the shoulders going to enter the brim? What is happening to the curve of Carus? Isn't it becoming a half circle?

Stretching and tightening of the large buttock muscles will stop the coccyx straightening, and increase the tension on the pelvic floor. Remember, all the muscles are at the back of the pelvis, and there is a good sized gap behind the pubes for the baby to descend through if he can get the back of his head into it.

At this stage the mother should be increasing the size of the pelvic outlet. Somehow, the idea took hold that lifting the legs equalled squatting. Well maybe the kind of squatting that Westerners can achieve, but that wasn't what was measured as increasing the outlet up to 30%. Those ladies were able to squat flat footed, with their thighs parallel to the floor, and s*wing their pelvis* forward as the baby descended. Their sacrum as well as their coccyx moved backward, as they arched their backs to allow the baby out.

The mother in bed, on her back is having things made as hard as possible. Her pelvis is curved upward and forward, increasing the pelvic floor resistance. The large muscles prevent the rhombus of Michaelis moving back as well as preventing the straightening of the coccyx.

Positions For Birth

How and where women give birth varies according to custom as well as to common sense. Most of the positions women are asked to adopt today have no basis in the latter, but have evolved to suit the professionals.

The supine position that is today's favoured position in Western hospitals is the one most likely to cause problems. We've looked at the effects of being bedridden, but if we want our colleagues to change their practise we need to be quite clear about the disadvantages.

During first stage labour, it is much simpler if the mother is mobile. All the uterine contraction pressure is available if she is able to bend forward with each pain. The baby has plenty of space between sacrum and pubes to tuck himself into the back of the pelvis.

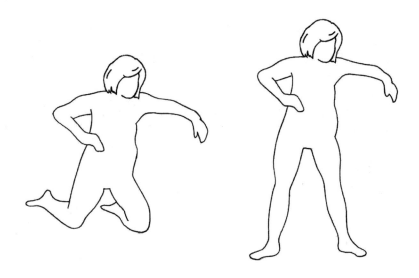

What's Wrong With Bed? Lots Of Things!!

- Firstly,once she's confined to bed, the mother's pelvis becomes an immobile tunnel, with all the accompanying difficulties. It might be all right if the tunnel was straight, but alas, it makes a 90° turn at the base of the cavity.

- Secondly most of the contraction force is wasted lifting the uterus and its contents before pressure can be applied to the cervix.

- Thirdly the mother is unable to change the internal pelvic measurements unless she has complete freedom to move her pelvis.

- Fourth the baby will have problems getting his head between the pubes and sacral prominence into the sacral curve, once the mother's legs are bent.

- If he does manage the above, he will have trouble lifting his head up and round the symphasis without lots of maternal pushing.

- Finally, he must now get his shoulders across the sacral prominence before he can get them into the pelvic cavity and rotate them.

When Bed Cannot Be Avoided

Left Lateral is the easiest birth angle for mothers confined to bed. It is also quite easy for the midwife, if she must help, to do so in this way;

- Stand beside or sit on the bed at the level of the mother's knees.
- Face her head.
- Allow her to reach up to the bedhead, or to hold onto her partner.

She will bend her legs, but rarely brings her knees close to her body. There is no need to lift the upper leg unless the mother wishes it.

She will arch her back with each contraction. As the baby is well forward on the abdominal muscles, and against the pubes, there may be little anal dilatation before the head begins to appear.

Some mothers throw their upper knee so far outwards that the sole of the upper foot is on the bed. This makes things awkward for the midwife, if she wants to "deliver" the baby rather than "catch" it. However, as long as the mother is able to lift her pelvis, there is rarely any problem.

If the baby should need his head flexed a little further, two fingers of the midwife's right hand on the muscles beside the perineum will help. Once his head is born, the baby will rotate in the usual fashion and bring its posterior shoulder out first. If the baby arrives behind the mother's body the midwife will need to pass it between the mother's legs as soon as it starts to breathe. There is plenty of length in the cord for this to be done before it is cut.

When the mother wants to give birth on her right side, things are a bit more complicated. We are used to working from the other side of the bed, but can adapt quite well when asked.

If the baby seems to be slow entering the direct A.P. diameter, a turn onto the mother's right side often hurries things along.

These positions can be used when the mother must be monitored throughout the birth. The I.V. is unrestricted, and the epidural catheter remains undisturbed. There is no need to disconnect the scalp electrode if one is in place. Abdominal monitoring is also feasible, though it's a good idea to experiment during early labour, until a routine that the midwife is comfortable with is devised.

Remember that the foetal heart should be heard moving progressively downwards and towards the middle of the maternal pubes, so the microphone does need to be adjusted frequently.

Very few babies have problems if their mothers are encouraged to avoid the dorsal posture.
Time enough for that when waiting for the placenta to be expelled.

Kneeling On The Bed

This position is a good one, but not over the head of the bed. -- that is fine during first stage, but not wise during second.

It may be difficult to persuade the mother to let her back sag towards the mattress as the baby descends. The sloping bedhead and the pile of pillows get in the way. The mother finds it easy to keep her hands on the mattress, instead of above her waist. Many women either keep their backs flat, or sometimes even rounded at this time. The chances of a tear are then much greater, as the pressure is into rather than in front of the pelvic floor. Many mothers sit back on their heels and push in this position, and that is even more likely if her hands are on the bed, making things worse.

Other problems start once the baby is born, and the mother tries to turn and sit on the bed. There is always some rubbish on the inco sheet under her knees, and often quite a pool of liquor and blood. Whether or not the mother is holding her baby, it is really hard to find a way to help her turn and change the bed as she does so. Often the first try is the last one.

The simplest way to handle a hands and knees birth on the bed, is to find an old fashioned nightingale (a sturdy bed table), arrange it at the end of the bed, and place a set of drawsheets and inco down there. If a few pillows are put on the table, the mother can spend most of her labour down there. The mother finds things better, as she will have her face not her bottom to the door. During second stage, her partner can stand at the bed end for her to hold him.

Once the baby is born, she tucks her toes under her and sits back against the pillows on a clean sheet at the top of the bed. Then, tidying the bed is simple.

143

It is much easier to again work from the "wrong" side of the bed. Whether the placenta is born before or after the move is up to those involved.

The first time a baby is seen being born at this angle is quite an experience! The face is at the midwife's waist level, and deciding how or where to touch the head is confusing.

Fortunately few of them need help, if the mother has allowed her spine to sag (the equivalent of arching it in other positions).

If not, the baby may need its head lifted slightly for a second or two to allow the shoulders to rotate. Some claim that tears are more common with this kind of birth, but if there is no rush, and the mother is free to move her hips that is not so.

The problems arise when the mother deliberately pushes with her back straight, or sits back on her heels. Once again, try to see that the posterior shoulder is born first.

If photos are taken with babies being born in this position, it is likely that the mother will want to destroy them once she has recovered. It is certainly an undignified posture, especially while just the head is born.

Supported Squatting and Birth Stools

Traditionally, women have given birth in some type of squatting position. In many societies, families had their own birth stool, or the midwife brought one. These, as can be seen in old pictures, had their seats at knee level, or a little higher.

Where life was simpler, women found places where they could find a rope or even a tree branch with which to support themselves.

As the baby descended, the mothers allowed their bodies to sag forward, and their knees to spread outwards. This provided the maximum space for the baby, and reduced the chance of tearing the perineum.

Today, many mothers wish to give birth in an upright, supported stance, which is easiest to provide when they have their feet on the floor. They can be held from behind, though when a contraction occurs, they will take their weight off their feet, and the supporter will have a "dead" weight to carry. Thus, the supporter should have a wall behind them to lean against. It is important to allow the knees to relax while holding the mother, or one's back can be damaged.

It is better to provide the mother with something sturdy to grasp---grab rails as provided for the elderly in showers or toilets are ideal.

Some have found holding on to the side of a birth pool or the kitchen worktop quite useful.

If nothing else is available, the mother may face her partner, and grasp him round the neck. This keeps the arms up, but has the disadvantage of restricting the mother's forward space.

145

Sometimes, the bed may be pulled out from the wall, and the mother can stand holding the bedhead.

At home, if they are well built, the stair rails may be useful, either alone or with a folded sheet, or something similar to pull on.

In fact, although there are many good and useful positions there is no one position for birth that suits all mothers.
All of the above should be discussed with impending mothers to allow them to consider the alternatives available <u>prior</u> to the onset of labour.

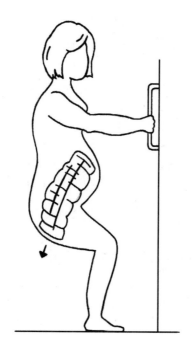

<u>An Upright, Supported Stance is helpful</u>

___Protocols – Be Creative! Be Aware!___

We need to find ways to complete the hospital records without disturbing the mother's labour rhythm.

Vital signs must be taken and recorded, but must it be within a couple of minutes before the couple has been given the chance to settle into a room?

Can they be done without the mother climbing into the bed? Once in, they are very hard to get out again.

Palpating the baby's position---can it be done with the mother standing? It feels odd the first few times, but if the mother tells us where she thinks the baby is lying, and we check with a portable sonic aid, they aren't hard to locate. The information is a lot more useful too.

Your unit demands a 30 minute cardiotocograph? Well, why can't Mum kneel on a squab on the floor, or over the top of the bed? What about kneeling over a beanbag, either on the floor or bed? Again, a lot more helpful, and definitely much less painful.

That admission vaginal exam---does it have to be done with the mother supine, or could she again be upright? It's surprising how much the relationships of the pelvic and foetal anatomy change when the mother lies on her back----it is not at all like when she is upright. It is also extremely uncomfortable, if not downright painful.

The mother with the baby presenting L O A is easily identified. Her protruding abdomen, swayback, duckwaddle walk, all tell us that she will do well. If she is encouraged to stay mobile, still with her knees lower than her seat--- (take a look at the chairs in the first stage area)

147

her labour should be short. If she is able to give birth in an upright position, whether on or off the bed, and her midwife does not insist on "delivering" her, her baby will be able to birth himself unaided.

We have seen how the normal process is meant to work. The mother responds to pressure from the baby's head by changing her posture to provide more internal space where it is needed.

If a midwife able to give her and her partner a private, safe environment, supports her, she will be able to enter the detached, endorphic state that allows good progress.

I know this isn't easy in a large unit, with so many people and activities to upset the balance. However, many places are making efforts to provide less interventions, and if research plus practical experience endorses the idea that properly prepared mothers need less "hands on" care, (and are therefore less of a burden to 'The Budget'), more will have to follow.

Pain Relief In Labour

Using the ideas in this book successfully, depends on co-operation between the birthing pair, and their care-giver. The mother needs to be able to feel what is happening inside her pelvis if she is to respond by increasing the available space. How are we to make sure that the pain is reduced as far as possible? Lets look at a few ideas

Water

The use of water for pain relief has become very popular. If it is used at home, the size of the hot water cylinder should be noted. There is no point in running out of hot water just as things get serious. Many mothers get great relief by standing in the shower with the water hitting their lower back. This also gets most of them leaning forward.

Ordinary baths are not much use during labour. First, it is hard to get enough water to cover the abdomen, and worse, the mother will be on her back. To be effective, she must kneel on all fours, and the base of the bath does not encourage her to stay like that. Maybe a sponge pad could be used to kneel on. One advantage is that she can lean on the side of the bath between contractions.

Spa pools, or transportable birth pools are fine, as they hold a lot of water---at home, check that the floor will be strong enough---and are either thermostatically controlled or can have more hot water added. The best are large enough for the mother to float on her abdomen. A six-person spa is perfect, and then the partner can also be in the water if desired. Whatever the size, it is important that again the mother keeps in forward leaning postures. Too many mothers sit on the shelf, and though the pain is reduced, there is no help for the uterus or baby .If the pool has soft sides, place a chair beside it for mother to lean on between contractions.

Whether the baby is born in the pool or outside is a matter of choice---it is important to think about how the mother will get out if she wants to. A few permanent pools are built into a platform onto which the mother can clamber with little effort---these are usually the spa kind with a seat right round that can be stood on. Lots of mothers just lean on the side and the midwife must reach behind them to catch the baby as it emerges.

Pethidine

Pethidine is often used, but once it is given, the mother cannot be mobile. It is extremely useful in very early labour if the baby has not fully rotated to the ideal L O A.

The mother is settled into a comfortable bed, on her left side, given an IM dose of 100mgs --or more if she is very large--and allowed to sleep. This has two effects. She will catch up on some of the sleep she has missed, and her muscles will really relax. If the baby does not turn, he is probably intending to stay where he is.

The most useful time to give pethidine seems to be to the mobile primigravida at around 9cm, as the overwhelming contractions of transition begin. A tiny dose - 12.5mg given I V will carry her through without any untoward effects.

Epidurals

Although these are so popular at present, they have several disadvantages. The need for an I V, the regular blood pressure checks and the continuous foetal monitoring are only a few. Epidurals are effective, in most cases, in relieving pain, but at what cost? We will ignore for now the controversial aspects, and think about how the labour itself is affected.

The absence of pain allows syntocinon to be used at a higher level than could otherwise be tolerated. It may have little deleterious effect on the uterus, but what about the baby? How is his head affected by the extra pressure?

Because the mother is really bedridden--trussed up by I V; monitor belt; B P cuff; epidural catheter; all needing her to keep still, and preferably remain on her back-- she is quite unable to help herself or her baby. This mother does have the totally immobile pelvis that causes so many problems.

How often do we think of placing the mother on her side, once the anaesthesia is effective? This would at least allow the baby more freedom, and avoid wasting so much of the contraction power. Maybe, we'd need only a fraction of the syntocinon to produce results.

Obviously, the mother would have to be turned from side to side at regular intervals to protect pressure points, but this could be done at "top up" times.

Epidurals And The Rhombus Of Michaelis

The rhombus of Michaelis, as we have seen, plays a very important role in allowing birth without pushing. As it moves backwards it pushes the ilia outwards also. Thus all diameters are increased by 1--2cm. Add the backward move by the coccyx, and it is easy to see where the extra space comes from, and why there is no need to push *an O.A.* baby out.

The action of the rhombus occurs only during physiological second stage labour. It appears to be triggered by the pressure from the back of the baby's neck on the nerve plexus at the junction of the bladder and urethra. It seems to correspond to the male prostate nerve supply. At least the reaction of the body is similar---the *foetal ejection reflex* described by Michel Odent.

When an epidural is in place what happens when second stage is reached, and the extra space should be provided? How can the rhombus move if its nerve supply is unable to function? Instead of a 16cm outlet, the baby, who is probably in a bad position anyway, must try and get out through 13cm. No wonder so many of them need pulling out!

If the mother is on her back, she is sitting on her sacrum instead of her ischial tuberosities so the baby must come down and around the symphasis, against the solid pelvic floor, rather than leaning against the pubes while he lifts his head.

The other unfortunate effect of an epidural is that the mother is unable to respond to pressure from the baby's head to increase the *available* space by shifting her weight, or lifting one or other leg. Thus the baby must be forced through a static tunnel, instead of twisting through a mobile space.

Induction and Augmentation

The modern idea of actively managing labour has consequences that need to be thought about.

There seem to be many more pregnancies going past term these days. If we look carefully at them, we see that most, if not all, are pregnancies where the baby is in an unsuitable position. He does not give his mother the proper signals and stimulus to cause her tissues to prepare for his birth. If a V.E. is done, the labia and vagina often feel like they should at 35 weeks, not 40.

The best thing that can happen is that the mother is shown how to help the baby to turn; but a few days are still needed to allow the maternal tissues to prepare.

Once induction has been decided upon, most units have a protocol for using prostaglandins. These mimic the normal hormones, but unfortunately tend to work only on the cervix. It becomes softer and dilatable, but the vagina and outlet have not relaxed.

The next step is usually ARM (artificial rupture of membranes) which almost guarantees that the baby will have problems turning to the right position.

It is also commonly forgotten that the tension inside the uterus drops dramatically once the liquor drains away, so contractions won't start until the uterine muscle has adapted. If they don't start as soon as the protocols demand, syntocinon augmentation is usually begun.

The action of syntocinon is not commonly studied by midwives, but it certainly should be. All it does, is make contractions stronger and more painful. It has no effect on the baby's position, which is causing the problem, or the flexibility of the maternal pelvis.

Because the contractions are far too close together, and too painful, the next step is an epidural for pain relief. Talk about iaterogenic or hospital induced problems!

Because the labour becomes even more unnatural, the foetal heart tracing becomes frightening, and a caesarian section is performed.

The baby arrives with Apgars of 9/1 10/5 10/10. Why? What is the first thing done when the decision to section is made? Yes, The syntocinon is turned off, and by the time he is extracted from the uterus, the baby has changed his blood several times, and is no longer at risk!! Crazy, but true.

The syntocinon packet insert used to state, "There shall be no more than three contractions, lasting 60 seconds or less in any ten -minute period. "How many units comply? Especially with primigravida ladies.

The time between contractions is needed by the baby in order to change his blood. During a contraction, the placenta is squeezed like a sponge. There is little or no blood flow. Once the contraction passes, the placenta must fill again, and the baby change his stale blood for fresh re-oxogenated blood.

All this takes time, and if the contractions are too close, is only partially completed. After 4 hours or so, the baby is really acidotic, especially if his mother has had no nourishment.

An electrolyte replacement I V drip should always be in place. There should be far fewer hypoglycaemic newborns if more thought was given to their needs during labour. They are pretty tough, but no one is indestructible.

Post Natal Pain Relief

When looking back on the birth of their baby, mothers frequently comment on how painful the episiotomy suture line has been. They also tell about the way their sex life has been upset by ongoing pain. This should not be such a problem.

If a mother has had an episiotomy, or nasty tear, that has been sutured, the aim is to prevent, or least reduce tissue swelling. Many places use ice packs, but not always effectively.

The most effective pack is a water filled, frozen fingercot, or maybe a condom. Obviously, the end is tied once it is filled. While suturing is being done, an assistant should bring 1 or 2 cots from the freezer, and wrap them securely in 2 opened gauze swabs.

As soon as the last stitch is in, place the pack *right on the suture line between the buttocks*. Now apply sanitary protection as usual. The packs are changed 1/2—1 hourly for a couple of hours, then discontinued.There will be virtually no swelling, so no tension on the tissues, and healing is much faster.

If the mother wishes, homeopathic Arnica 6 or 30 given 1/2 hourly for 3-4 doses will also help.

Section Eight

Ideas For Those Times When Things "Go Wrong"

Section Eight: Ideas For Those Times
When Things "Go Wrong"

*" The mother was unperturbed by the whole event, but
the midwife felt she needed
a medicinal brandy! "*

Shoulder Dystocia

This is apparently becoming more common during the past few
years. The average baby may be a little larger, but even small ones
are causing trouble. It seems to be yet another consequence of
delivery in bed and in the dorsal position. It is also very likely to
happen to some degree when the "Rest and be Thankful" stage is
omitted.

Think of the 3450g baby whose mother pushes ineffectually for an
hour, and then is "rescued" by a ventouse delivery. The shoulders
failing to finish rotating at the brim were all that stopped it being
born.

Avoidance is the best policy, fairly easy if the mother is mobile and
keeps her pelvis thrust forward during the actual birth. This action
allows the movement of the rhombus, increasing the space at the
brim, in the cavity and at the outlet, and keeps the baby in the best
position for shoulder rotation.

It is important to understand that *while the anterior shoulder is seen
first, the posterior shoulder must be born first.* Why it was ever

changed is unclear. The top of the anterior shoulder uses the maternal symphasis as a fulcrum on which to swing the baby's body downward while the weight of the head pulls it forward. Thus there is nothing to impede the birth of the posterior shoulder. No pressure on the perineum at any stage.

However, most of us want to know what to do when the shoulders are already stuck. They are most likely still in the oblique at the brim, and unable to enter the pelvis until they are directly transverse. Rotation to the direct anterior /posterior angle takes place once they are far enough into the cavity to be below the sacral prominence.

The mother is almost certainly on her back with knees up. Check which side the baby's back is on by noting the way he is trying to turn. If he's L. O. A. it will be towards the mother's right thigh. If an R O A it will be towards her left.

First; get the legs down. Help the mother to turn onto her side. The right for an L O A, the left for an R O A.

Ask the mother to arch her back. If she can't or won't as sometimes happens, stand at her back and push her bottom away from you, or ask a support person on the other side of the bed to pull her towards him/her. This alone may be enough. If not, check that the mother's knees are further down the bed than her seat. Now ask the mother to raise her upper leg. This increases the useable space in the pelvis, and allows the baby space to turn.

Next look to see if the anterior shoulder is visible (don't be too worried about the congested face). If not bring the head slightly backwards until you can see the junction of the shoulder and neck. Sometimes the rotation is not complete even after all this moving, so be sure it is.

Now move the head towards the mother's abdomen, thus placing the flat top of the shoulder against the inside of the symphasis, and the neck in the outlet, with the bulk of the body lying directly anterior/ posterior in the cavity and allow the posterior shoulder to emerge.

Some midwives prefer to have the mother on hands and knees in the knee-chest position, which also works if she will let her back sag towards the bed and keep her knees as far as possible behind her bottom--that is, the spine and thighs are at an angle of around 120°. The leg on the same side as the baby's back should be raised, and the sole of the foot placed on the bed or floor. The key is to be sure that the anterior shoulder stays inside and against the symphasis until the posterior is out.

Again, when the mother has been actively pushing in a deep squat, (not a good idea), the baby may be unable to rotate its shoulders. If the mother is helped to stand, and then adopt an all-fours posture with the knee supported, there will be room for the baby to turn. Sometimes the wrong knee is chosen and the mother must move again. The leg will be the one on the same side as the baby's back. She is increasing the available space in the brim and cavity of the pelvis.

Whichever method is tried, remember;

- The mother must create as much space as possible between her spine and pubic bone, whichever position she is birthing in.

- The head enters the pelvis in the transverse, and rotates to the direct anterior/ posterior position in order to pass the spines and emerge. As it turns, the shoulders become transverse, and slide into the cavity, where they in turn rotate to the direct anterior/posterior position to pass the spines, as the head turns to face its original direction.

If time has been allowed between first and second stage labour for the uterus to regain its tone and the baby to finish his rotation, there will seldom be a second stage lasting more than 30 minutes.

When women gave birth in the left lateral position, shoulder dystocia was almost unknown. It is the action of raising the legs and bringing the symphasis and spine close together, and asking mothers to push just because they are "fully dilated" that causes almost all delays in second stage, or shoulder dystocia.

Mary's Story

Mary, Gravida 4 / Para 3 has been in labour for some time with a largish baby.

Her midwife is a firm believer in the squatting position for giving birth. Mary has several helpers, two of whom are kneeling beside her providing support. Her baby's head is finally out, but nothing more happens.

After quite a time, and a lot of effort, Mary decides that there is no way her baby will be out unless she moves. She tries to stand, but her helpers are in the way, so she subsides onto all fours, with her right knee on one friend's upper leg. Several strong pushes, but no change. Mary tries again, and this time it is her left knee on the other helper's thigh.

Movement!! What a relief!

She can feel the baby coming down. She drops her spine and gives the "primal scream" (written about by Michel Odent) and the baby emerges. Despite the long time its head had been born, the baby had Apgars of 8 & 10.

Another Experience – Karen's Story

Karen had laboured on her hands and knees while leaning against the sofa. First stage went slowly, and second stage seemed to last forever.

Eventually a large head appeared, and almost at once looked as if it was trying to go back (the classic "turtle" action). She tried pushing even harder, but nothing happened. Then she tried raising first one leg for several contractions and then the other.

Eventually, she almost stood up, and the baby was born. What a congested face he had.

The reason that he was unable to emerge was that Karen was far too close to the sofa. Her seat was level with her ankles so her pelvis and spine were too close together. Once she got her knees right back and the angle between body and legs open there was plenty of room.

Meconium Aspiration

This is one of the things that we have been taught to fear. It can be a problem for the midwife with no other professional help at hand. The danger of aspiration and subsequent pneumonia is all too real. However, like most things, once the normal sequence of events immediately after birth is reviewed, we see that preventive action is available.

The first thing to be aware of is that there is no emergency until the cord stops pulsating. So, leave baby attached to his mother. The baby should be face down if he has come out unaided. If not, turn him that way.

Using your right hand, palm against his chest wall, thumb under his right arm and fingers along his left chest wall, and lift him till his face is lower than his waist.

Hold him quite firmly, as the idea is to prevent him breathing ***until he has sneezed***. This usually happens spontaneously, but if not a tickle of the end of his nose works. Any meconium that has not drained out will be sneezed out and then all is well.

Trying to clear the airway and handle everything else unaided will take years off any midwife's life. It may also be damaging to the baby.

Donna's Story

This one caught everyone napping. In a small unit, only one midwife on duty, with a Nurse/aide to help, there were six mothers and another gravida 3/ para 2 in labour.
Everything seemed to be going well, and the midwife went off to answer the phone and order the stores. Suddenly there was a call from the birth room, where the mother had reached full dilation extremely quickly. The midwife found her lying back, membranes ruptured, with the baby in a pool of heavily meconium stained liquor between her legs. From around 5cm to birth in ten minutes!!

Father rang the bell for more help --ie. someone to ring the doctor, while the midwife picked the baby up in her hand and hung him to drain. Copious fluid drained from his nose and mouth, but his cord was still beating well.

The baby was also rather shocked from his precipitate arrival so was covered with a warm towel.

Before the doctor arrived (he had to come from the surgery some distance away) the baby had sneezed several times so was allowed to take a breath, still face down. No more drainage was seen so the cord was clamped and cut as part of the normal routine.

From then on there was nothing to show just what a close thing his birth had been. He might well have taken an early breath, and inhaled much of the pool he was lying in. Fortunately this did not happen.

His mother however, needed treating for shock. Blood loss was minimal, but the speed of the birth had allowed her system no time to adapt.

Prolapsed Cord

How dangerous this is, depends on many factors. It is always frightening though, and help needs to be sought at once.

Whether at home, in a Birth Centre, or in hospital, if it occurs in early labour, then the baby's head must be held off the cervix until the obstetrician intervenes. That is, the mother is placed in the knee-chest posture, and the midwife pushes the baby upwards internally. If contractions are strong, and the mother is not in hospital, ask if an asthma inhaler can be used.-three good puffs will often slow things down long enough to reach effective help but a medical practitioner must order this.

If it happens during second stage, then it depends whether the mother is a primigravida or multigravida. It is more serious in the first case, as her perineum still has to stretch, so if possible the baby must again be held up till help is available. This is not easy in an ambulance, and very difficult in a car!

When the baby of a multigravida ruptures its membranes on the pelvic floor, and a cord is seen, it _may_ be safer to send for help and then ask the mother to grasp her support person, arch her back, and push.

Saying firmly "GIVE ME THE BABY NOW " usually works. Once is enough. If it's not out, then it must again be kept off the pelvic floor.

Fortunately, it's a very rare emergency, as most cords float.

Sue's Story

Sue was progressing well with her first labour. She was in a mid-sized unit, and it was around 3am. All her records were good, so no one was expecting what happened.

At full dilation, with her baby still just at the spines, there was a sudden gush of liquor, and, horrors, a loop of cord!!

There was no way the baby could be born quickly enough, before he had squashed his cord and been lost. Things happened amazingly fast. The obstetrician was rung and wakened at home, some distance away. The midwife sat on the bed and held the baby off the pelvic floor with a gloved hand. Her assistant was relieving in another area of the hospital, (serving supper!) so how she did things is guesswork.

Somehow she reached the forceps, and had things ready by the time the obstetrician arrived. There was no time for a pudendal block, or even a local to work, so Sue puffed on the entonox as the forceps were applied to the baby. A quick twist, a firm pull, and he was out!

It was a demonstration of fast thinking and action, by experts. A pity there was no one to appreciate it. (No, it had nothing to do with me.)

The assistant returned to find the perineal tear being repaired and the baby perfectly happy on his mother's abdomen. If a caesarian had been needed it would have been much longer before the theatre staff were available, so it was fortunate that two such experienced people were involved.

Diane's Story – Multigravida

Diane was having her second baby at home.

Her first birth had been uneventful--a six hour labour, no tears or episiotomy. This birth was proceeding quickly. All records fine, membranes intact.

First stage ended, and as full dilation was reached the membranes ruptured.

Clear liquor, but what's this? A loop of cord too. The midwife promptly arranged for a transfer to hospital for an emergency caesarian. She didn't ask Diane to try to push the baby out while waiting to move, but pushed the baby up off the pelvic floor.

The transfer was successful, and Diane's baby was born by L.S.C.S within minutes of their arrival at hospital. Everyone was fine. In this case, with the baby very low in the pelvis, a good push would probably have seen him out--maybe a tear, but well worth a try.

Unfortunately, the baby was quite slow reaching her milestones, and by two was well behind her contemporaries.

Maybe she would always have been slow, but there would have been nothing to lose in asking her mother to try and push her out.

Cord Round The Neck More Than Once

Some babies, while practising gymnastics in the womb, manage to wrap their cords round their necks more than once. This is a serious state, as there is more chance of them being unable to move down even when the uterus has shrunk. They may also be more likely to suffer oxygen shortage as the cord stretches.

Many of them show signs of unhappiness that are picked on the monitor tracing, or with the sonic aid. Some are plain even with a fundascope. Some give no real clues except that they fail to descend as fast as they should. It would be very helpful if, when late pregnancy scans are done, the position of the baby's cord was noted. Just once round the neck or the body is seldom a problem, but any more means that the possibility of having to cut the cord before the baby is fully born is much more likely. This also creates an emergency if the baby is slow to breathe.

The art of midwifery involves preventing emergencies wherever possible.

Trisha's Story

Trisha was happily getting on with having her baby. This was a much wanted "late baby", but Trisha had had four others with no difficulty. This one seemed the same. Trisha was upright, and relatively mobile.
All the records were fine, but the midwife was unhappy. What was she missing? This baby would give her trouble she felt.

The only thing apparent was that the baby didn't appear to be descending. Still, that's not uncommon in some racial groups---full dilation, ruptured membranes, and a baby from abdomen through the pelvis all in one spectacular move are their norm. Trisha was from such a group.

Time passed, and finally Trisha felt like pushing. Must have been pressure from the "waters" as the baby was too high to exert any pressure.

The head began to appear, the ears were born and then – nothing!

Trisha pushed hard, changed position, and tried some more.

The G P was rung but the baby needed to be born before he had time to arrive. Finally, the midwife slipped her fingers up beside the baby's head to see what could be felt. A very tightly wound cord, maybe more than one loop?

Somehow, two forceps were applied to the same loop of cord. The scissors were slipped into the gap between the forceps, and the cord cut, while the midwife prayed hard.

Working without knowing what was wrong, and totally out of sight was frightening.

A forcep was lifted and the cord unwound. Three loops! Still no descent!!

The other forcep was lifted, and unwound in the opposite direction. Two more loops!! This was unbelievable!

Now the G P arrived and said, "It's better to leave cutting the cord till the baby is born".

The midwife replied, "We'd all feel better if you turned the resus table on please".

During this exchange, the baby slid into the bed, opened her eyes and began to breathe!! A quick check, and she was declared fine. She had been a very lucky baby - not many can manage to wrap their cord five times round their neck and live through their birth!

The mother had been unperturbed by the whole event, but the midwife felt she needed a medicinal brandy!

There had been no way that this baby could have been moved through the loops of cord, or pushed up out of the way.

The really interesting thing was that the midwife had been so sure that a problem would be present, even though all the records said otherwise.

Gut feelings are often right.

Obviously, the dorsal or left lateral positions had been the only ones for this birth.

Section Nine

Changing The Culture

Section Nine: Changing The Culture

"Ingenuity had to be used to find ways to conform to protocols, whilst encouraging independence of thought and action by the birthing family."

<u>How It Worked In Real Life.</u>

For an eleven-year period, the author was able to incorporate the practises discussed in this book into her working environment. This was on an informal basis. It occurred gradually over a period of time by teaching antenatal classes, and sharing in as many parent contact situations as possible.

The idea that there was a grand design for human birth, that if followed gave good results, became increasingly part of the district's philosophy. The whole community must accept the idea for things to change from a dream to reality. It took 3 years before the idea of labouring out of bed to become routine - 3 years!!! The best and most enduring changes often take the longest time to come into effect. Patience, as they say, is a virtue.

Also the unit had been designed when only women, staff and doctors were allowed into the birthing area, and doors were placed so that several rooms could be viewed at once either from the corridor or while "delivering" a baby just by turning one's body. Hardly conducive to mothers removing their clothes, or doing anything but cowering on the bed. Brown paper and glue came in handy. Then curtains were eventually used to encourage people to "knock" before entering rooms.

Getting women off their backs, and to start with, into left lateral for birth was equally slow.

Then the idea of kneeling over a beanbag became popular---- especially if it was on the floor, or the mother was facing the door.

Actually getting the bed moved to a position that allowed reasonable privacy was difficult, as the gas and oxygen, suction, telephone, electrical outlets etc. were in the wrong places.

Ingenuity had to be used to find ways to conform to protocols whilst encouraging independence of thought and action by the birthing family.

A great deal of effort went into teaching the concept of Optimal Foetal Positioning---though at this stage the name had not been coined. Many partners were either farmers or engineers, so they happily became involved in understanding the foundation facts on which the actions depended.

Eventually, the transfer in labour rate dropped from around 35% to 5%, and the forceps rate from the previous 4-5 monthly (on top of the transfers) to 2-3 per year. The forceps in their long life packs spent more time travelling to be resterilised than being used!

Another eye-opener was the sudden difference in the number of primigravida ladies with babies in the correct position when waterbeds first appeared. How did they work? Well, the first ones were like overgrown hot water bottles. When Dad got into bed, the water moved over to Mum's side. She settled down, with her abdomen relaxed into the warmth, and her baby snuggled himself into the back forward position. Thus she was still able to sleep on her left side and these babies were well prepared for their birth. They didn't need much help to get themselves into a position from which they were able to trigger off labour and follow the classic path described in all our books.

Then mothers were helped to form small groups that met regularly, but informally, and the amount of mutual help increased. Mothers were taught to check urine and weight (if still recorded). They followed the baby's growth on a graph, and as he grew bigger, worked out his position. Taking the maternal blood pressure did remain part of each visit. Abdominal palpations continued, though only to conform to protocols in most cases.

Discussion among mothers as they waited to be seen---the problem was to keep them away--helped emphasise the shape of their abdomen, and the baby's position was talked about regularly. The normality of many minor hassles was also shared and a midwife was always about to clear up any niggling questions.

Mothers who had problems understanding such things as scan comments, or unsure how baby was settling, were able to drop in and discuss their worries almost any morning between 11am and midday.

Taking part in Parents Centre classes became routine, as did Friday morning hospital classes. Finally, after talking about Normal Birth at classes and visits for 5 years we had achieved the 85% normal, 5 % transfer to base, results. A primigravida was expected to give birth in less than 8 hours from starting labour, and a multigravida in less than 3hours. (The discrepancy covers those mothers who needed specialist care in a base hospital. They became steadily fewer, as the knowledge spread among professionals and clients.).

Any mother who had not made significant progress in 4 hours of one-on-one help was transferred, as there was little chance that the situation would resolve. This meant that we had a peaceable lifestyle, with very few dramas, and a happy postnatal group. Mothers who were comfortable, very few sutures, no haemorrhoids, and babies full of the pleasure of being born. It was easy to establish real bonding.

As with so many of these small units we were finally closed in the interests of "efficiency" and "economies of scale".

Postnatal care – Then and Now

For centuries women who were menstruating, or who had just given birth were segregated from the community. Their duties, especially if they involved food, were taken over by other women of the family or tribe.

This had the major benefit of giving women a rest from their arduous life. It also allowed women time to spend with a new baby, getting to know it and establishing a breastfeeding habit.

As the industrial age developed and large cities developed, families lived in separate houses, and women continued their normal duties during their periods. Even when babies were born there was little time to rest.

This century, mothers were allowed to "lie in" for several days while a young girl did the daily chores. Later, women went to hospital for around two weeks before returning home to take up full care of the house and family. Though they loved this, it had a major downside.

Whilst in hospital mothers were not even allowed to visit the toilet! Meals were taken in bed; babies were brought out to feed; nappies already changed.

The real damage was done by the few bedpans given each day. Whether the post partum diuresis was considered unimportant, or not known about I have no idea, but women had seriously distended bladders, and by the time they rose from bed their pelvic floors had no strength. Inevitably they went home to lifting and carrying, everything from wood to water and washing and all things between, and their pelvic floors sagged slowly towards their knees.

Obviously the doctors were kept busy surgically repairing the damage. They decided that the problem was that "heads are left on the perineum far too long, and are damaging the pelvic floor." Episiotomies were encouraged to avoid this, and only now are we realising that in most cases there is no need to do one.

Today we have swung to the opposite end of the spectrum. Mothers are expected to be super women, and be resuming normal life and back at work within weeks. No one seems to see that for many women birth is no longer a safe simple family event, but a surgical operation. Mothers have one intervention after another until so many are trying to deal with an anaesthetic, an operation and a baby.

These mothers really need help at home for several weeks to allow time for complete recovery. Unfortunately, their female relations will also be working and unable to help. Teenage girls are in full time education today, when once they would have helped with the household and the new baby.

We can't turn the clock back but we must find a way to give expectant and new mothers the support they need.

Can The Culture Be Changed ?

The answer, of course, is yes. History bears witness to the fact that protocols and traditions surrounding birth have changed.

Often there have been "swings of the pendulum" first in one direction and then, ironically, in the complete opposite direction.

It can be done. I know. I've done it.

We do however need to understand the birth process thoroughly ourselves and allow that knowledge to motivate and propel us to action.

This motivation needs to be coupled with a strong determination and a good dose of courage if we are to work within the "system's" current limitations and eventually bear witness ourselves to the welcome difference that keeping "the normal" normal will make to *everybody.*

Patience will also be a very useful quality if we are to gently but confidently communicate this "almost lost" knowledge of old. Remember – there is nothing new in these pages. Just forgotten.

It is my sincere hope and prayer that in writing this book I will have gone some way towards injecting that dose of understanding and motivation necessary to generate renewed determination within this honourable profession of midwifery to do the job we first entered the profession to do!

Section Ten

A Final Look

Section Ten: A Final Look

"If we all work together, we may be able to leave our current blind alley that is reducing birth to a surgical procedure."

As we've travelled through this book, it has been my hope that many everyday situations have become clearer.

Throughout mankind's existence the midwife has been the expert in caring for birthing families. She passed her knowledge to her apprentices on the job, and in most cases the system worked well. Unfortunately, as reproduction became a political interest, and religious practises controlling it became widespread, the midwife was found to be a dangerous wise woman.

Originally, in almost all societies, midwives were recruited from women whose own families were grown up. During the recent past, this has changed as the medical rather than the midwifery model has gained sway.

Birth is now controlled by obstetricians, and midwives have been trained more as obstetric nurses in most countries. Once giving birth in hospital, and the large ante-natal clinics became the norm, the chance to really know the families was lost.

The idea of controlling the time, place and type of birth that she would have seems to have been accepted by mothers without any real research being done. Pregnant women are usually fairly docile and easily manipulated by caregivers. We all know how using the words, "It is better for the baby" defuses resistance. How often can we honestly say it?

The best thing for the baby is to teach his mother about the one designed way of birth, and help her achieve it. In only one type of birth do all the factors, maternal and foetal, work together to achieve the safest, simplest, shortest, birth possible.

Giving birth requires that physical, hormonal, and emotional ingredients function smoothly and at the correct time. Throughout the pregnancy, the baby has been changing his mother's body to suit his needs. Birth is one of the automatic processes, just the same as digestion. It's in, and the body knows what to do with it.

Enough preaching!

To finish this off we'll have a quick look at the factors needed for a straightforward birth.

The mother makes sure that from 35/40 weeks, **at all times** she keeps her knees lower than her seat, and her abdomen lower than her spine. This keeps the pelvic inlet open, and forms a hammock of the abdominal muscles.

This baby is most comfortable lying vertex L O A, so he will assume this position, and have no problems engaging his head. He will give good signals to ripen his mother's body ready to let him out, and he will be born close to term.

The baby lying vertex R O P is the one who, if not shifted, will need help.

Let's now briefly review the recommendations I have made in the previous chapters of this little book.

There are three places to intervene.

1. *Ante-natally*

Ante-natally, by teaching the mother and her support people about the importance of Optimal Foetal Positioning. Once the key points are understood, most families do their best to help themselves.

They need to know:

- That Braxton Hicks contractions have no effect on changing the baby's position.
- That the mother must keep her weight above or in front of her ischial tuberosities,
- That she must sleep on her left side, using a thin pillow to support her abdomen if the upper muscles get sore.
- That the pregnancy lordosis is essential, so it is better to wear a girdle than to tuck the tail under.

2. *First Stage Labour*

In early labour

When the baby has failed to engage, and contractions are long, strong and too close from the beginning, the baby's head will be unable to bend under the sacral prominence, and his back will be upright. The idea is to get his bottom well forward and persuade him to rotate.

If the baby is still facing forward and the membranes are intact (highly unlikely) the mother should try walking up and down a flight of stairs. Going up and down sideways is even better. If she is at home, or out of the public eye, she could crawl up and walk down which often works well. It is not a race, she is changing the oblique diameters of her pelvis with each stair, and giving the baby more space. This is often effective if done while awaiting induction.

Pacing the corridors is a waste of time and energy.

If protocols allow, a small meal, a substantial dose of pain relief --- Pethidine, morphine--- and a good sleep will often be enough.
If induced, or augmented, labouring in a kneeling position or abdomen down over a beanbag is good.

Later in labour

If the baby has failed to rotate, and progress is slow, then as soon as it is possible for the midwife to insert two fingers into the cervix and part them---around 5cm is easiest--she should do so. Ask the mother to kneel on the bed, leaning over the top. Sit on the bed, and insert two fingers into the vagina. Rest the elbow of the right arm on the bed, and allow the baby to be pushed down by the next contraction. It will turn either immediately, or by the third contraction if it is going to.

This procedure is very uncomfortable, so three contractions is enough. The reason for the hands and knees position is that unless the baby's shoulders turn he will fall back into the O P position within a few minutes.

3. *Second Stage*

Many mothers get to full dilatation of the cervix, and then despite strong pushing fail to progress.

Maybe the *"Rest and be Thankful"* stage has been forgotten.

The need to push shows that the baby is not positioned correctly.

A short pause may allow him time to finish turning. If not, then check to see that his shoulders are transverse. If not, which way should they turn?

The mother may need to lie on her right side for a couple of contractions to help him move. Then again upright, with knees wide apart and leaning forward while he brings his head down may be the right move.

Remember, he must get his posterior shoulder to lead, and to do this, it must get below the sacral prominence.

If at all times, the mother has her weight in front of her ischial tuberosities, she will move her pelvis at the baby's urging. Then he will be born without any need to push. He will come out, posterior shoulder first, and lie face down on whatever solid base his mother is on.

Birth should and can be a fulfilling, empowering experience for mothers, and a safe journey for baby if all the rules of the blueprint are followed. This requires all those involved in helping and supporting birthing families to deeply understand the process.

Once we internalise the knowledge of what a comprehensive self regulating process pregnancy and birth is, we will be able to focus on ways to bring as many situations as possible back to the normal, and recognise early those which are unable to be influenced.

Knowing when serious intervention is needed and being able to access that help is important.

Maybe in years to come, when the importance of the baby's role has been acknowledged, all the old ideas will be thoroughly researched and become mainstream care.

If we all work together, we may be able to leave our current blind alley that is reducing birth to a surgical procedure. Birth will become what it is meant to be; a safe, simple awe-inspiring everyday miracle.

Our babies, having had their heads protected in O A labours, will be as bright, peaceful and happy, as I am sure they should be.

Many of the so-called minor physical, emotional and mental difficulties will be things of the past, and more and more children will fulfil the wonderful potential they have been born with.

Midwives and Antenatal Teachers are the people who can pioneer the "new" teaching, and, as it appears to be an idea whose time has come, will find a receptive audience among birthing families.

I wish you success for the sake of our next unborn generation.

Jean Sutton 2001

About The Author

Jean Sutton - NZ RGON Reg. Midwife, Cert. Adult Education

New Zealand born, Jean is a mother and grandmother, with four grown-up children and five grandchildren. She is also a midwife with a long-established family background in farming and engineering.

Her working life began at 17 years of age, when she became a nurse-aid in a rural maternity hospital. Here she witnessed over 200 babies born with only one forceps delivery in a year! Birthing was a totally normal process to the young Jean Sutton, who had seen many calves, lambs, foals and piglets born with seldom any outside intervention whatsoever!

Jean went on to train as a general nurse, but her love of birthing meant that she continued to work in maternity hospitals after she qualified.

Pausing only to give birth and raise a family herself, Jean never forgot the lessons she had learned thus far. It was during this period that several of her own extended family had the most appalling birth experiences which were quite an anomaly to Jean. These essentially motivated her to return to her career and resume her training, becoming a qualified midwife. During the period in which she continued to train she was amazed to see that the "normal" birthing process had become increasingly rare; more and more babies were being "helped" into this world. What was going wrong?

Combining knowledge gained from having been involved with

normal birthing processes almost all her life and already understanding the relationship between the maternal pelvis and the foetal head from an engineering perspective, Jean began to dig deeper. Her observations, gleaned from detailed anatomical studies and research from old midwifery textbooks, have led her to develop the pioneering concept known as OPTIMAL FOETAL POSITIONING.

In 1980 Jean became Principal Nurse / Midwife of a small country maternity hospital. During her 11 years in this position Jean was able to implement her discoveries. The intervention rate during this period dramatically dropped from over 40% to 10%.

Now convinced these are long lost principles that need to be taught, from her base in New Zealand Jean travels the world, passionately sharing the concepts that undergird OFP.

Her first book, "Understanding and Teaching Optimal Foetal Positioning" (co-written with Pauline Scott) has helped numerous women to enjoy the God-given miracle of straightforward birth. Selling thousands of copies in over 40 countries, Jean is now increasingly in demand internationally as a speaker at conferences and study days.

Interested in Booking a Study Day with Jean Sutton?

Please contact Julie Sutton at:

julie@birthconcepts.freeserve.co.uk

or write to:

**Julie Sutton
95 Beech Rd
Bedfont TW14 8AJ
United Kingdom**

For a full Organiser's Pack including booking terms and conditions.

Please state preferred month, year and location for the booking.

ALL FEEDBACK WELCOME!

Jean will be very pleased to receive any comments and queries resulting from the reading of this book.

Although she cannot guarantee to answer all feedback personally, comments will be warmly received and where possible a reply will be given.

Please address all correspondence to the publishers:

**BIRTH CONCEPTS UK
95 BEECH RD
BEDFONT TW14 8AJ
UNITED KINGDOM**